Lecture Notes in Computer Science 10594

Commenced Publication in 1973
Founding and Former Series Editors:
Gerhard Goos, Juris Hartmanis, and Jan van Leeuwen

More information about this series at http://www.springer.com/series/7409

Siuly Siuly · Zhisheng Huang
Uwe Aickelin · Rui Zhou
Hua Wang · Yanchun Zhang
Stanislav Klimenko (Eds.)

Health
Information Science

6th International Conference, HIS 2017
Moscow, Russia, October 7–9, 2017
Proceedings

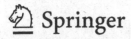 Springer

Editors
Siuly Siuly
Centre for Applied Informatics
Victoria University
Melbourne, VIC
Australia

Zhisheng Huang
Vrije University of Amsterdam
Amsterdam
The Netherlands

Uwe Aickelin
University of Nottingham
Nottingham
UK

Rui Zhou
Swinburne University of Technology
Melbourne, VIC
Australia

Hua Wang
Victoria University
Melbourne, VIC
Australia

Yanchun Zhang
Victoria University
Melbourne, VIC
Australia

Stanislav Klimenko
Institute for High Energy Physics
Protvino
Russia

ISSN 0302-9743   ISSN 1611-3349 (electronic)
Lecture Notes in Computer Science
ISBN 978-3-319-69181-7   ISBN 978-3-319-69182-4 (eBook)
https://doi.org/10.1007/978-3-319-69182-4

Library of Congress Control Number: 2017956087

LNCS Sublibrary: SL3 – Information Systems and Applications, incl. Internet/Web, and HCI

Printed on acid-free paper

This Springer imprint is published by Springer Nature
The registered company is Springer International Publishing AG
The registered company address is: Gewerbestrasse 11, 6330 Cham, Switzerland

Preface

The International Conference Series on Health Information Science (HIS) provides a forum for disseminating and exchanging multidisciplinary research results in computer science/information technology and health science and services. It covers all aspects of health information sciences and systems that support health information management and health service delivery.

The 6th International Conference on Health Information Science (HIS 2017) was held in Moscow, Russia, during October 7–9, 2017. Founded in April 2012 as the International Conference on Health Information Science and Their Applications, the conference continues to grow to include an ever broader scope of activities. The main goal of these events is to provide international scientific forums for researchers to exchange new ideas in a number of fields that interact in-depth through discussions with their peers from around the world. The scope of the conference includes: (1) medical/health/biomedicine information resources, such as patient medical records, devices and equipment, software and tools to capture, store, retrieve, process, analyze, and optimize the use of information in the health domain; (2) data management, data mining, and knowledge discovery, all of which play a key role in decision-making, management of public health, examination of standards, privacy and security issues; (3) computer visualization and artificial intelligence for computer-aided diagnosis; and (4) development of new architectures and applications for health information systems.

The conference solicited and gathered technical research submissions related to all aspects of the conference scope. All the submitted papers in the proceedings were peer reviewed by at least three international experts drawn from the Program Committee. After the rigorous peer-review process, a total of 11 full papers and seven short papers among 44 submissions were selected on the basis of originality, significance, and clarity and were accepted for publication in the proceedings. The authors were from eight countries, including Australia, Bulgaria, China, Colombia, Japan, Pakistan, Russia, and The Netherlands. Some authors were invited to submit extended versions of their papers to a special issue of the *Health Information Science and System* journal, published by BioMed Central (Springer).

The high quality of the program – guaranteed by the presence of an unparalleled number of internationally recognized top experts – can be assessed when reading the contents of the proceedings. The conference was therefore a unique event, where attendees were able to appreciate the latest results in their field of expertise, and to acquire additional knowledge in other fields. The program was structured to favor interactions among attendees coming from many different horizons, scientifically and geographically, from academia and from industry.

We would like to sincerely thank our keynote and invited speaker:

- Professor James Jhing-fa Wang, President, Tajen University, Pingtung, Taiwan and Chair Professor, National Cheng Kung University, Tainan, Taiwan

Our thanks also go to the host organization, Moscow Institute of Physics and Technology, Russia. Finally, we acknowledge all those who contributed to the success of HIS 2017 but whose names are not listed here.

October 2017   Siuly Siuly
                                                          Zhisheng Huang
                                                            Uwe Aickelin
                                                               Rui Zhou
                                                               Hua Wang
                                                         Yanchun Zhang
                                                    Stanislav V. Klimenko

Organization

General Co-chairs

Stanislav V. Klimenko   Moscow Institute of Physics and Technology, Russia
Yanchun Zhang   Victoria University, Australia and Fudan University,
             China

Program Co-chairs

Siuly Siuly   Victoria University, Australia
Zhisheng Huang   Vrije Universiteit Amsterdam, The Netherlands
Uwe Aickelin   The University of Nottingham, UK

Conference Organization Chair

Hua Wang   Victoria University, Australia

Publicity Co-chairs

Grazziela Figueredo   The University of Nottingham, UK
Yan Li   University of Southern Queensland, Australia

Publication and Website Chair

Rui Zhou   Swinburne University of Technology, Australia

Local Arrangements Chair

Maria Berberova   Moscow Institute of Physics and Technology, Russia

Webmasters

Jiannan Li   The University of Adelaide, Australia
Weikang Wang   The University of Adelaide, Australia

Program Committee

Omer Faruk Alçin   Bingöl University, Turkey
Varuṇ Bajaj   Indian Institute of Information Technology, Design
             and Manufacturing, Jabalpur, India
Mathias Baumert   The University of Adelaide, Australia
Jiang Bian   University of Florida, USA

Contents

Software for Full-Color 3D Reconstruction of the Biological Tissues Internal Structure

A.V. Khoperskov[1](✉) ⓘ, M.E. Kovalev[1] ⓘ, A.S. Astakhov[1,2](✉) ⓘ,
V.V. Novochadov[3](✉) ⓘ, A.A. Terpilovskiy[4] ⓘ, K.P. Tiras[5] ⓘ, and D.A. Malanin[6] ⓘ

[1] Institute of Mathematics and Information Technologies, Volgograd State University, Volgograd, Russia
{khoperskov,a.s.astahov}@volsu.ru
[2] Institute of Computing for Physics and Technology, Protvino, Moscow Oblast, Russia
[3] Institute of Natural Sciences, Volgograd State University, Volgograd, Russia
biobio@volsu.ru
[4] The Laboratory of Virtual Biology Ltd., Moscow, Russia
[5] Institute of Theoretical and Experimental Biophysics of RAS, Moscow, Russia
[6] Volgograd State Medical University, Volgograd, Russia

Abstract. A software for processing sets of full-color images of biological tissue histological sections is developed. We used histological sections obtained by the method of high-precision layer-by-layer grinding of frozen biological tissues. The software allows restoring the image of the tissue for an arbitrary cross-section of the tissue sample. Thus, our method is designed to create a full-color 3D reconstruction of the biological tissue structure. The resolution of 3D reconstruction is determined by the quality of the initial histological sections. The newly developed technology available to us provides a resolution of up to 5–10 μm in three dimensions.

Keywords: Scientific software · Computer graphics · 3D reconstruction · Biological tissues · Image processing

1 Introduction

Different approaches and methods of 3D-visualization of biological tissues are discussed depending on the scientific goals and objectives of practical applications [1, 2, 14]. A significant number of software complexes, libraries and specialized systems of scientific and technological visualization for three-dimensional digital biomedicine have been developed [7, 9, 12, 24, 25]. Approaches using medical X-ray tomography are very effective for 3D-reconstruction of tissues/organs [8]. We can also highlight some areas that are associated with the localization of implanted biomaterials [8, 26], the colonoscopy, the ultrasonic sounding [9], the stereoscopic fluorescence imaging, the multispectral magnetic resonance image analysis [16], the single photon emission computed tomography (CT) [11], the electron tomography [6], the use of combined methods [9]. The transition begins from micro-CT to nano-CT [8, 20].

This work is addressed to the anatomical or destructive tomography (biotomy) approach [17, 23]. A newly developed method is based on making of a set of high-quality

© Springer International Publishing AG 2017
S. Siuly et al. (Eds.): HIS 2017, LNCS 10594, pp. 1–10, 2017.
https://doi.org/10.1007/978-3-319-69182-4_1

images of biological tissue histological sections using the high-precision grinding of a pre-frozen biological sample [22].

The advantages of the proposed approach:

- A high-quality photography offering all the benefits of the raster graphics.
- A realistic color rendering.
- Very high accuracy up to several microns.
- Absence of "screening interference" in contrast to non-destructive methods [26].
- High speed access to information about individual fragments of the tissue.

The main disadvantage of the proposed method is principle impossibility of living tissue usage due to its physical destruction during the process of preparation of a set of images slices. Another disadvantage of the method associates with utilization of digital raster photographs. 3D modeling can improve the efficiency of various solving aims tasks, including endoprosthetics [5, 8, 10, 15, 26, 27].

2   Making of an Images Set of Histological Sections

The process of producing of images set includes the following steps (Fig. 1):

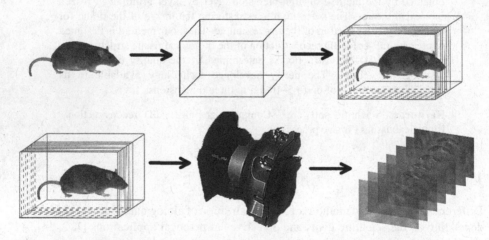

Fig. 1.   The sequence of steps for making of an images set of biological tissue histological sections

1. Selection of a biological object in accordance with the objectives of the study.
2. A formation of the original sample by fixing a biological object by a casting material in a three-dimensional mold.
3. The original sample of the biological object is rapidly frozen in the form of a rectangular parallelepiped. The fixation of the biological object is ensured by at cryogenic temperatures (T $\leq$ –72 °C), after that it is filled by the casting material (at T $\leq$ –25 °C) [19].
4. The sample is placed into a special device for layer-by-layer grinding.

5. An optical system adjustment is required due to the sample thickness change as a result of layer-by-layer removing.
6. Visual analysis of the images allows distinguishing photos with a blurred focus, highly modified illumination and other optical artifacts (removing images of poor quality if it is necessary).

As a result, we have an ordered snapshot sequence of biological tissue slices with step Δz, whose resolution determined by sample size and used object-glass. The Δx and Δy resolution of the equipment available at The Laboratory of Virtual Biology, Ltd. is 6–20 μm, while the Δz resolution is 5–20 μm.

3 Creation of Θ-Sections and Software Development

Let us introduce a Θ-rectangle ("theta-rectangle") to denote a rectangle inscribed into the polygon of the sample section. Various ways of Θ-rectangle specification in a triangular section are shown in Fig. 2.

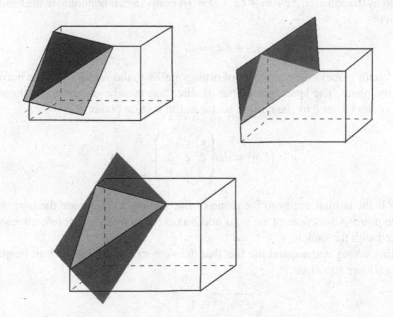

Fig. 2. The examples of the Θ-rectangles in a triangular section

Hereafter the RGB color system is applied. Each element of the mapping color table P is considered like a vector in the three-dimensional space. Thereby, within the closure region of the sample space the vector field $\vec{\Omega}(x, y, z) = \{R, G, B\}$ is a set that converts it into a color space. To construct an image on the sample slice plane, the Θ-rectangle of this section have to be divided into pixels. Each pixel is associated with a color depending on its spatial position in a vector field $\vec{\Omega}$.

A set of slices images is the initial data

$$z_k = (k - 1)\Delta z, \tag{1}$$

where the k-th image number ($k = 1, ..., M$) is determined by the z-coordinate of the histological section.

The sample vertex in the upper left corner of its frontal face relatively to the camera location during the record is taken as origin. Let us Consider a numbered set of raster images (1) of size $P_x \times P_y$, where P_x and P_y are the numbers of pixels for the two corresponding sides. Such an initial set of images is also called a digital set of base slices.

To reconstruct an object in the form of a three-dimensional model, a method for color interpolation in the space between each adjoining pair of images in the plains z_k and z_{k+1} should be specified. The entire set of initial images is considered as a three-dimensional matrix $\hat{P} = (i, j, k)$, whose elements are individual pixels of images from the set. Their addressing is determined by the number of the k-th layer (a sequence number of a photo), the number of the i-th row and the number of the j-th column in the matrix of pixels of the k-th photo. We have used discrete functions defined on a three-dimensional grid (x_i, y_j, z_k).

The statement that the vector ξ is orthogonal to the normal vector to the plane described by the equation $Ax + By + Cz + D = 0$ is equivalent tantamount to the following expression:

$$A\xi_x + C\xi_z = 0. \tag{2}$$

The vector η obeys the conditions of orthogonality to the vector ξ and the normal to the section plane. The latter means that its direction may be computed as the vector product of the vector ξ by the normal vector to the section plane:

$$\eta = [\xi, n] = det\begin{pmatrix} e_x & e_y & e_z \\ \xi_x & \xi_y & \xi_z \\ A & B & C \end{pmatrix}, \tag{3}$$

where n is the normal vector to the plane of the section, e_x, e_y, e_z are the unit vectors along the positive directions of the x-, y- and z-axes respectively in the reference system associated with the sample.

Finally, taking into account the fact that the vectors ξ and η have a unit length, we obtain two more equations:

$$\sqrt{\xi_x^2 + \xi_z^2} = 1, \tag{4}$$

$$\sqrt{\eta_x^2 + \eta_y^2 + \eta_z^2} = 1. \tag{5}$$

From Eqs. (2–5), we can calculate the coordinate values for the vectors ξ and η:

$$\xi = \left\{ \frac{C}{\sqrt{A^2 + C^2}}, 0, -\frac{A}{A^2 + C^2} \right\}, \tag{6}$$

$$\eta = \left\{ -\frac{AB}{L}, \frac{A^2 + C^2}{L}, -\frac{BC}{L} \right\}, \tag{7}$$

$$L = \sqrt{A^2 B^2 + (A^2 + C^2)^2 + B^2 C^2}. \tag{8}$$

To solve the problem of the long time required a data reading from the hard disk, we choose a special basis on the plane of the section. We denote by p, q the unit vectors along the directions of the abscissa and ordinate axes, respectively, in the reference system associated with the section plane. Thus, the vector p is orthogonal to the unit vector directed along the applicate axis in the reference system associated with the sample:

$$p_z = 0, \tag{9}$$

where p_z is the projection of the vector p onto the given axis.

Moreover, it is required adding equations denoting the orthogonality of the vector p to the normal vector to the plane of the section, and the orthogonality of the vector q to both of them, as well as the condition that the length of the vectors p and q is equal to one. Accounting for all the listed above conditions we obtain the following equations:

$$A p_x + B p_y = 0, \tag{10}$$

$$q = det \begin{pmatrix} e_x & e_y & e_z \\ p_x & p_y & p_z \\ A & B & C \end{pmatrix}, \tag{11}$$

$$\sqrt{p_x^2 + p_y^2} = 1, \tag{12}$$

$$\sqrt{q_x^2 + q_y^2 + q_z^2} = 1. \tag{13}$$

From the Eqs. (9–13), we can determine the values of the coordinates of the basis vectors in the reference system associated with the sample:

$$p = \left\{ -\frac{B}{\sqrt{A^2 + B^2}}, \frac{A}{\sqrt{A^2 + B^2}}, 0 \right\}, \tag{14}$$

$$q = \left\{ -\frac{AC}{M}, -\frac{BC}{M}, \frac{A^2 + B^2}{M} \right\}, \tag{15}$$

$$M = \sqrt{A^2 C^2 + B^2 C^2 + (A^2 + B^2)}. \tag{16}$$

The Eqs. (14) and (15) specify the directions of the basis vectors of such reference system, associated with the cross-section plane, for which the natural order of pixel bypass would guarantee the optimal number of calls to information recorded on the hard disk.

4   Examples of Images Reconstruction in Arbitrary Sections

A human knee-joint ($20 \times 10 \times 10$ cm in 20 μm steps) and a rat knee-joints (with a pixel size of 8×8 μm and a pitch of 8 μm) are considered as an examples of the section constructions. The samples were obtains in compliance with all legal norms. These sets could be easily identified by color of casting material. Green and red filling correspond to the rat and human knee-joints, respectively.

Images of different shapes of sections are considered below. If the section does not have the shape of a rectangle, then the image is supplemented with a black background (no restriction on the background color) (Figs. 3, 4, 5 and 6).

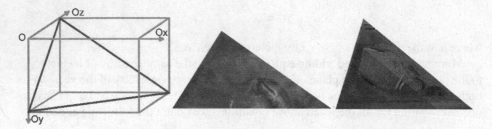

Fig. 3. Triangular sections

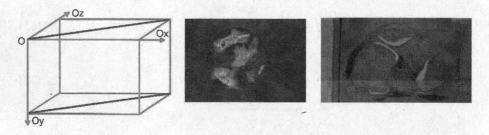

Fig. 4. Cross-sections with 4 angles

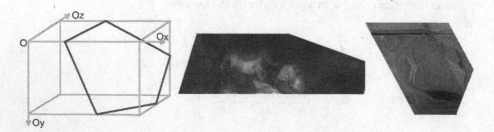

Fig. 5. Cross-sections with 5 angles

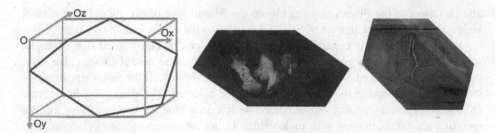

Fig. 6. Cross-sections with 6 angles

5 Information System for Modeling

The developed software package includes two main parts: programs with a graphical user interface (GUI) and calculation modules (DLL) for modeling user-defined slices. Microsoft Visual Studio 2012 comprising C# programming language with .NET framework 4.5 has been utilized as the software development environment. The programming interface is refined by API WPF. User selects a folder with input data, sets the geometric parameters of the sample (length, width, height and step Δz as seen from Fig. 7) and sections (three points along which the plane will be built). The file names are determined by the section number in the sequence.

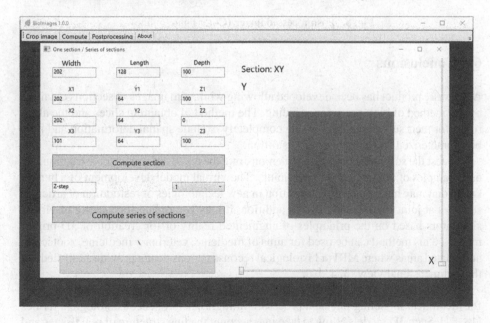

Fig. 7. Setting of an arbitrary slice

After the previously described actions with the help of calculation modules, the program creates an object of the Cuboid class (with the specified length, width and depth) and an object of the Plane class describing the frontal face of the cuboid (the normal vector is co-directed with the OZ axis and applied to the origin - (0, 0, 0)).

Beside the one slide calculation, series of slices can be constructed (for example, series of images with a given step in the range 1–6°). In the case if images size vary, they should be enlarged to the same size. In order to do this all the resulting slices are analyzed and the image with the largest width is selected. The remaining images are enlarged to chosen size and supplemented with a gray-blue background (Fig. 8). The resulting images are marked with angle values. Using the images movie can be compiled (for example, for XY- and XZ- sections (along the Z- and Y- axes, respectively)).

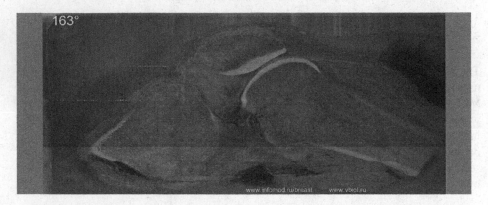

Fig. 8. Postprocessed image (Color figure online)

6   Conclusions

A software product has been developed allowing work with images of sections obtained by the method of high-precision grinding. The method of obtaining slices and the algorithm for their subsequent processing completely exclude spatial deformation and may be characterized by minimal color distortion.

To test the software complex and demonstrate the results of section construction, we used samples of human and rat knee-joints. The virtual model development of a human knee-joint may have practical application in new technologies of restoration of articular surfaces at joint injuries [17, 18]. In addition, it may be applied for making of virtual simulators based on the principles of augmented reality or for creation of 3D-printer models. This method can be used for aims of medicine, veterinary medicine, zootechny and related areas where MRI or histological reconstructions do not provide a full-fledged three-dimensional view [3, 4, 10].

We can use this method to construct vector 3D models of samples that are necessary for theoretical modeling physical processes in highly heterogeneous biological tissues [18, 21]. Such 3D models allow to take into account the fine structure of real tissues and changes in their physical parameters. The joint use of image processing techniques and numerical modeling methods such as computational fluid dynamics or heat transfer is a modern trend in the development of medicine and applied biology [13].

Acknowledgments. KAV and AAS are thankful to the Ministry of Education and Science of the Russian Federation (project No. 2.852.2017/4.6). NVV thanks the RFBR grant and Volgograd Region Administration (No. 15-47-02642).

References

1. Azinfar, L., Ravanfar, M., Wang, Y., Zhang, K., Duan, D., Yao, G.: High resolution imaging of the fibrous microstructure in bovine common carotid artery using optical polarization tractography. J. Biophotonics **10**, 231–241 (2017). doi:10.1002/jbio.201500229
2. Bobroff, V., Chen, H.-H., Delugin, M., Javerzat, S., Petibois, C.: Quantitative IR microscopy and spectromics open the way to 3D digital pathology. J. Biophotonics **10**, 598–606 (2017). doi:10.1002/jbio.201600051
3. Brazina, D., Fojtik, R., Rombova, Z.: 3D visualization in teaching anatomy. Procedia Soc. Behav. Sci. **143**, 367–371 (2014). doi:10.1016/j.sbspro.2014.07.496
4. Candemir, S., Jaeger, S., Antani, S., Bagci, U., Folio, L.R., Xu, Z., Thoma, G.: Atlas-based rib-bone detection in chest X-rays. Comput. Med. Imaging Graph. **51**, 32–39 (2016). doi: 10.1016/j.compmedimag.2016.04.002
5. Cerveri, P., Manzotti, A., Confalonieri, N., Baroni, G.: Automating the design of resection guides specific to patient anatomy in knee replacement surgery by enhanced 3D curvature and surface modeling of distal femur shape models. Comput. Med. Imaging Graph. **38**(8), 664–674 (2014). doi:10.1016/j.compmedimag.2014.09.001
6. Chen, Y., Wang, Z., Li, L., Wan, X., Sun, F., Zhang, F.: A fully automatic geometric parameters determining method for electron tomography. In: Cai, Z., Daescu, O., Li, M. (eds.) ISBRA 2017. LNCS, vol. 10330, pp. 385–389. Springer, Cham (2017). doi: 10.1007/978-3-319-59575-7_39
7. Chiorean, L.D., Szasz, T., Vaida, M.F., Voina, A.: 3D reconstruction and volume computing in medical imaging. Acta Technica Napocensis **52**(3), 18–24 (2011)
8. Cuijpers, V.M.J.I., Walboomers, X.F., Jansen, J.A.: Three-dimensional localization of implanted biomaterials in anatomical and histological specimens using combined x-ray computed tomography and three-dimensional surface reconstruction: a technical note. Tissue Eng. Part C Methods **16**, 63–69 (2010). doi:10.1089/ten.TEC.2008.0604
9. Ermilov, S.A., Su, R., Conjusteau, A., Anis, F., Nadvoretskiy, V., Anastasio, M.A., Oraevsky, A.A.: Three-dimensional optoacoustic and laser-induced ultrasound tomography system for preclinical research in mice: design and phantom validation. Ultrason. Imaging **38**, 77–95 (2016). doi:10.1177/0161734615591163
10. Ha, J.F., Morrison, R.J., Green, G.E., Zopf, D.A.: Computer-aided design and 3-dimensional printing for costal cartilage simulation of airway graft carving. Otolaryngol. Head Neck Surg. 1–4 (2017). doi:10.1177/0194599817697048
11. Hanney, M.B., Hillel, P.G., Scott, A.D., Lorenz, E.: Half-body single photon emission computed tomography with resolution recovery for the evaluation of metastatic bone disease: implementation into routine clinical service. Nuclear Med. Commun. **38**, 623–628 (2017). doi:10.1097/MNM.0000000000000686
12. Ioakemidou, F., Ericson, F., Spuhler, J., Olwal, A., Forsslund, J., Jansson, J., Pysander, E.-L.S., Hoffman, J.: Gestural 3D interaction with a beating heart: simulation, visualization and interaction. In: Proceedings of SIGRAD 2011, KTH, Stockholm, pp. 93–97 (2011)
13. Ko, Z.Y.G., Mehta, K., Jamil, M., Yap, C.H., Chen, N.: A method to study the hemodynamics of chicken embryo's aortic arches using optical coherence tomography. J. Biophotonics **10**, 353–359 (2017). doi:10.1002/jbio.201600119

14. Lee, R.C., Darling, C.L., Staninec, M., Ragadio, A., Fried, D.: Activity assessment of root caries lesions with thermal and near-IR imaging methods. J. Biophotonics **10**, 433–445 (2017). doi:10.1002/jbio.201500333

15. Mohammed, I.M., Tatineni, J., Cadd, B., Gibson, I.: Advanced auricular prosthesis development by 3D modelling and multi-material printing. In: Proceedings of the International Conference on Design and Technology. DesTech Conference, Geelong, pp. 37–43 (2017). doi:10.18502/keg.v2i2.593

16. Murino, L., Granata, D., Carfora, M.F., Selvan, S.E., Alfano, B., Amato, U., La-robina, M.: Evaluation of supervised methods for the classification of major tissues and sub-cortical structures in multispectral brain magnetic resonance images. Comput. Med. Imaging Graph. **38**(5), 337–347 (2014). doi:10.1016/j.compmedimag.2014.03.003

17. Novochadov, V.V., Khoperskov, A.V., Terpilovskiy, A.A., Malanin, D.A., Tiras, K.P., Kovalev, M.E., Astakhov, A.S.: Virtual full-color three-dimensional reconstruction of human knee joint by the digitization of serial layer-by-layer grinding. In: Mathematical Biology and Bioinformatics. Reports of the VI International Conference, Puschino, pp. 76–78 (2016)

18. Novochadov, V.V., Shiroky, A.A., Khoperskov, A.V., Losev, A.G.: Comparative modeling the thermal transfer in tissues with volume pathological focuses and tissue engineering constructs: a pilot study. Eur. J. Mol. Biotechnol. **14**, 125–138 (2016). doi:10.13187/ejmb.2016.14.125

19. Novochadov, V.V., Terpilovsky, A.A., Shirokiy, A.A., Tiras, K.P., Klimenko, A.S., Klimenko, S.V.: Visual analytics based on recoding input color information in 3D-reconstructions of human bones and joint. In: C-IoT-VRTerro 2016, pp. 257–260. Institute of Physical and Technical Informatics, Protvino (2016)

20. Papantoniou, I., Sonnaert, M., Geris, L., Luyten, F.P., Schrooten, J., Kerck-hofs, G.: Three-dimensional characterization of tissue-engineered constructs by contrast-enhanced nanofocus computed tomography. Tissue Eng. Part C Methods **20**, 177–187 (2014). doi:10.1089/ten.TEC.2013.0041

21. Polyakov, M.V., Khoperskov, A.V.: Mathematical modeling of radiation fields in biological tissues: the definition of the brightness temperature for the diagnosis. Sci. J. VolSU Math. Phys. **5**(36), 73–84 (2016). doi:10.15688/jvolsu1.2016.5.7

22. Terpilovskij, A.A., Kuz'min, A.L., Lukashkina, R.A.: Method for creating a virtual model of a biological object and a device for its implementation. Patent of the Russian Federation. Invention No. 2418316, 10 May 2011. Bull. 13

23. Terpilovskiy, A.A., Tiras, K.P., Khoperskov, A.V., Novochadov, V.V.: The possibilities of full-color three-dimensional reconstruction of biological objects by the method of layer-by-layer overlapping: knee joint of a rat. Sci. J. Volgograd State Univ. Nat. Sci. **4**, 6–14 (2015). doi:10.15688/jvolsu11.2015.4.1

24. Turlapov, V.E., Gavrilov, N.I.: 3D scientific visualization and geometric modeling in digital biomedicine. Sci. Vis. **7**(4), 27–43 (2015)

25. Uma Vetri Selvi, G., Nadarajan, R.: A rapid compression technique for 4-D functional MRI images using data rearrangement and modified binary array techniques. Australas. Phys. Eng. Sci. Med. **38**, 731–742 (2015). doi:10.1007/s13246-015-0385-y

26. Weber, L., Langer, M., Tavella, S., Ruggiu, A., Peyrin, F.: Quantitative evaluation of regularized phase retrieval algorithms on bone scaffolds seeded with bone cells. Phys. Med. Biol. **61**, 215–231 (2016). doi:10.1088/0031-9155/61/9/N215

27. Xu, X., Chen, X., Li, F., Zheng, X., Wang, Q., Sun, G., Zhang, J., Xu, B.: Effectiveness of endoscopic surgery for supratentorial hypertensive intracerebral hemorrhage: a comparison with craniotomy. J. Neurosurg. 1–7 (2017). doi:10.3171/2016.10.JNS161589

Epileptic Seizure Detection Using EEGs Based on Kernel Radius of Intrinsic Mode Functions

Qiang Li, Meina Ye, Jiang-Ling Song, and Rui Zhang$^{(\boxtimes)}$

The Medical Big Data Research Center, Northwest University, Xi'an, China
{lqlq,yemeina,sjl}@stumail.nwu.edu.cn, rzhang@nwu.edu.cn

Abstract. The study of automated epileptic seizure detection using EEGs has attracted more and more researchers in these decades. How to extract appropriate features in EEGs, which can be applied to differentiate non-seizure EEG from seizure EEG, is considered to be crucial in the successful realization. In this work, we proposed a novel kernel-radius-based feature extraction method from the perspective of nonlinear dynamics analysis. The given EEG signal is first decomposed into different numbers of intrinsic mode functions (IMFs) adaptively by using empirical mode decomposition. Then the three-dimensional phase space representation (3D-PSR) is reconstructed for each IMF according to the time delay method. At last, the kernel radius of the corresponding 3D-PSR is defined, which aims to characterize the concentration degree of all the points in 3D-PSR. With the extracted feature KRF, we employ extreme learning machine and support vector machine as the classifiers to achieve the task of the automate epileptic seizure detection. Performances of the proposed method are finally verified on the Bonn EEG database.

Keywords: Automatic seizure detection · Electroencephalogram (EEG) · Empirical mode decomposition (EMD) · Phase space representation (PSR) · Kernel-radius-based feature · Extreme learning machine (ELM) · Support vector machine (SVM)

1 Introduction

Epilepsy is a serious chronic neurological disorders that has an active incidence of 4–8/1000 and may affect both children and adults [3]. It is characterized by periodic and unpredictable occurrence of seizures, which are resulted from abnormal discharges of excessive amount of brain neurons, and usually appears to be the muscle stiffness, staring and impaired consciousness etc. [6].

As an electrophysiological monitoring approach to record electrical activities of the brain, electroencephalogram (EEG) has been widely applied in clinics due to its potential for exploring the physiological and pathological information in the brain. For epilepsy patients, the seizure detection using EEGs becomes an important and necessary step in the diagnosis and treatment. However, the traditional seizure detection by a trained neurologist always appears costly and

© Springer International Publishing AG 2017
S. Siuly et al. (Eds.): HIS 2017, LNCS 10594, pp. 11–21, 2017.
https://doi.org/10.1007/978-3-319-69182-4_2

inefficient, as well as sometimes includes subjective factors. Therefore, issues regarding the automatic seizure detection have been raised by more and more researchers in these decades. In order to realize it successfully, extracting proper features from EEG signals, which are then fed into a classifier so that the epileptic EEGs can be distinguished from background EEGs, is acknowledged to be one of the key points.

Since it has been demonstrated that human brain is a nonlinear dynamical system, the application of various nonlinear analysis methods for extracting features from EEGs presents a new avenue to exploit the underlying physiological processes. With the recognition that the system in non-seizure periods is more complex comparing with that in seizure periods, fractal dimension [20], sample entropy [16], permutation entropy [11], correlation sum [17] and recurrence quantification analysis (RQA) [2] have been explored to be the extracted features. Differently, in accordance with the similarity analysis, dynamical similarity index [13], fuzzy similarity index [12] and Bhattacharyya-based dissimilarity index [9], have been proposed to find the transition from a seizure-free state to a seizure state. If a non-seizure EEG segment is defined as the reference template, then the less similar a given present EEG segment is with the template, the more possible it will be the epileptic one. Originated from the fact that the anti-persistence of systems in non-seizure periods is weaker than that in seizure periods, various extraction methods on the basis of detrended fluctuation analysis index and Hurst exponent have been designed in [19]. Meanwhile, from the chaoticity analysis point of view, the Lyapunov exponent of EEG signals has also been taken as the feature for completing the seizure detection in [18]. Furthermore, given an EEG signal, the distribution uniformity and scatter degree of its lagged *Poincaŕe* plot have been presented in [15], which are defined to measure the difference between seizure EEGs and non-seizure EEGs intuitively.

In this study, a new kernel-radius-based feature (KRF) extraction method is proposed, where the kernel radius of three-dimensional phase space representation (3D-PSR) of an intrinsic mode function (IMF) is defined to be the feature. The key idea can be summarized as follows. Due to the fact that small change in EEG signals may be amplified when signals are decomposed and analyzed on smaller frequency-bands separately [10], the given EEG signal is first decomposed into different numbers of IMFs adaptively by using the empirical mode decomposition (EMD) method. Then the 3D-PSR is reconstructed for each IMF according to the time delay method. Next, kernel radius of the corresponding 3D-PSR is defined, which aims to characterize the concentration degree of all the points in 3D-PSR. With the extracted KRF, we finally apply support vector machine (SVM) and extreme learning machine (ELM) to achieve the task of epileptic seizure detection automatically.

The remainder of this paper is organized as follows. Section 2 systematically describe the proposed feature extraction method. Section 3 introduces the EEG database and discusses the experimental results, and some remarks are concluded in the last section.

2 Methods

2.1 Empirical Mode Decomposition

Empirical mode decomposition (EMD), which is a fundamental part of the Hilbert Huang Transform (HHT), has been proposed for analyzing non-linear and non-stationary signals by Huang et al. [5]. Applying EMD, a complicated signal can be decomposed into a finite and often small number of components. Such components, which are named as intrinsic mode functions (IMFs), constitute a complete and almost orthogonal basis of the original signal.

An IMF is defined as a function satisfying two conditions: (i) there holds $|a - b| \leq 1$ where a and b denote the numbers of extrema and zero-crossings of the signal; (ii) there holds $\frac{e_+ + e_-}{2} = 0$ at any point where e_+ and e_- represent two envelopes of the signal. The iterative process of extracting IMFs from the given signal can be summarized in the following algorithm [8].

Algorithm I (EMD): Given a signal $\mathbf{s} = \{s(t)\}_{t=1}^{N}$.

Step 1. Identify the local maxima and local minima from $s(t)$ respectively.

Step 2. Construct the upper envelope $e_+(t)$ and lower envelope $e_-(t)$ of $s(t)$ by using the cubic spline interpolation.

Step 3. Calculate the mean of $e_+(t)$ and $e_-(t)$, which is denoted by

$$m(t) = \frac{e_+(t) + e_-(t)}{2}.$$

Step 4. Extract $h(t)$ from $s(t)$ as

$$h(t) = s(t) - m(t).$$

Step 5. If $h(t)$ satisfies two conditions for IMF, then stop; otherwise, let $s(t) = h(t)$ and repeat steps 1–5 until $h(t)$ satisfies the conditions. According to EMD, the original signal $s(t)$ can be represented by

$$s(t) = \sum_{i=1}^{M} X_i(t) + r(t), \ t = 1, 2, \cdots, N. \tag{1}$$

Here, $X_i(t)$ denotes the ith IMF, $r(t)$ denotes the residual and M is the number of IMFs of $s(t)$, which is determined by the method adaptively.

Figure 1(a) and (b) illustrate the IMFs of a non-seizure EEG segment and a seizure EEG segment respectively.

2.2 Kernel-Radius-Based Feature Extraction Method

For each IMF, we reconstruct its phase space by time delay method [4]. In our work, we have confined our discussion to the value of embedding dimension as three, because of its visualization simplicity and performance reliability.

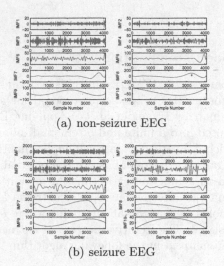

(a) non-seizure EEG

(b) seizure EEG

Fig. 1. IMFs of EEG signals decomposed by EMD

We name the corresponding plot as the 3-dimensional phase space representation (3D-PSR) in what follows.

Denote by $\mathbf{X}_i = \{X_i(1), X_i(2), \cdots, X_i(N)\}$ the ith IMF, we then construct its 3D-PSR as

$$\mathbf{Y_i} = \{Y_i^{(k)} : k = 1, 2, \cdots, N - 2\tau\}$$

where

$$Y_i^{(k)} = [X_i(k), X_i(k + \tau), X_i(k + 2\tau)]^T,$$
$$k = 1, 2, \cdots, N - 2\tau.$$

For visualization, we write $P_i^{(k)}$ to denote the corresponding point of $Y_i^{(k)}$ in the 3D phase space, and $\mathbf{PSR}_i = \{P_i^{(k)} : k = 1, 2, \cdots, N - 2\tau\}$ the collection of all points in terms of $\mathbf{X}_i$. Figure 2 illustrates the 3D-PSR plots of non-seizure EEG and seizure EEG respectively.

It can be easily seen from Fig. 2 that the points in 3D-PSR of seizure EEG distribute more sparse than those of non-seizure EEG. Therefore, we focus on characterizing the concentration degree of the points in $\mathbf{PSR}_i$ to be the extracted feature, which can be then applied to discriminate the seizure EEGs from non-seizure EEGs.

Firstly, we define the center $O_i = (a_i, b_i, c_i)$ of $\mathbf{PSR}_i$ according to the following way:

$$a_i = \frac{1}{N - 2\tau} \sum_{k=1}^{N-2\tau} X_i(k),$$

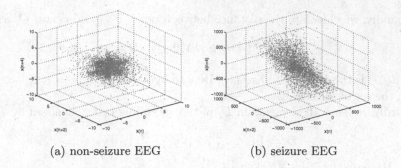

(a) non-seizure EEG   (b) seizure EEG

Fig. 2. The 3D-PSRs of IMF_1 corresponding to the non-seizure EEG and seizure EEG

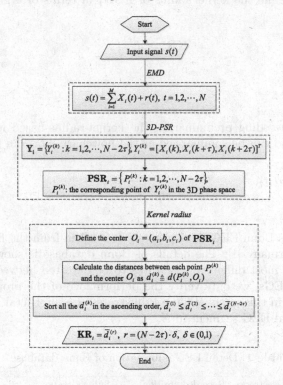

Fig. 3. The flowchart of KFR feature extraction method

$$b_i = \frac{1}{N - 2\tau} \sum_{k=1}^{N-2\tau} X_i(k + \tau),$$

$$c_i = \frac{1}{N - 2\tau} \sum_{k=1}^{N-2\tau} X_i(k + 2\tau).$$

Secondly, we calculate the distance between point $P_i^{(k)}$ and center O_i as

$$d_i^{(k)} \triangleq d(P_i^{(k)}, O_i), k = 1, 2, \cdots, N - 2\tau$$

where $d(\cdot, \cdot)$ is the Euclidean distance. Denote by $D_i = \{d_i^{(k)} : k = 1, 2, \cdots, N - 2\tau\}$ be the set of all distances.

Thirdly, we sort all elements in D_i in the ascending order, denoted by

$$D_i = \{\bar{d}_i^{(1)}, \bar{d}_i^{(2)}, \cdots, \bar{d}_i^{(N-2\tau)}\},$$

where $\bar{d}_i^{(1)} \leq \bar{d}_i^{(2)} \leq \cdots \leq \bar{d}_i^{(N-2\tau)}$.

Finally, we define the kernel radius of $\mathbf{PSR}_i$ in terms of a given threshold $\delta \in (0, 1)$ to be

$$\mathbf{KR}_i = \bar{d}_i^{(r)}$$

where

$$r = (N - 2\tau) \cdot \delta.$$

With the proceeding preliminaries, the kernel-radius-based feature (KRF) extraction method can be summarized as the flowchart shown in Fig. 3.

3   Experiments

3.1   Database

This work applies Bonn EEG database, which is taken from the Department of Epileptology, Germany [1]. The details of Bonn database is shown in Table 1. Because it is the most difficult for seizures to be detected between ictal EEGs and inter-ictal EEGs, we only verify the performance of the proposed method on sets D and E in this paper. Figure 4 illustrates one inter-ictal EEG segment in D and one ictal EEG segment in E.

Table 1. Detail EEG information of Bonn database

Data set	Recording electrodes	Recorded position	Subject state
A	Scalp electrode	Cortex	Awake and relaxed state with eye open of five healthy people
B	Scalp electrode	Cortex	Awake and relaxed state with eye closed of five healthy people
C	Intracranial electrode	Hippocampal formation	Period of inter-ictal of epilepsy patients
D	Intracranial electrode	Epileptogenic zone	Period of inter-ictal of epilepsy patients
E	Intracranial electrode	Epileptogenic zone	Period of ictal of epilepsy patients

[1]Each data-set comprises 100 epochs of single-channel EEG signal, which are 23.6 s single-channel EEG signals with 173.61 HZ sampling rate.
[2]There is no artifact in all EEGs.

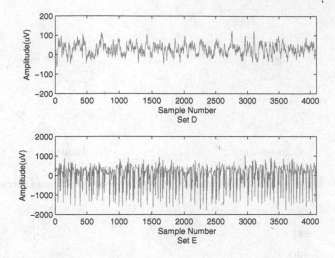

Fig. 4. Sample EEG recordings in set D (inter-ictal) and set E (ictal)

Table 2. Specified parameter in the experiments

Methods	Parameter	Symbol	Specified values
ELM	Number of hidden nodes	L	10
SVM	Regularization parameter	C	2^{-5}
SVM	Kernel width	g	2^{-6}
Kernel radius	Threshold parameter	δ	0.5

3.2   The Experimental Results and Discussions

This subsection will verify the performance of the proposed automated seizure detection method, which combines the kernel-radius-based feature (KRF) with extreme learning machine (ELM) and support vector machine (SVM) respectively.

In ELM, the additive hidden nodes $G(\mathbf{a}, b, \mathbf{x}) = g(\mathbf{a} \cdot \mathbf{x} + b)$ are applied and the optimal number of hidden nodes is determined by ten-fold cross validation. Here, $(\mathbf{a}, b)$ are weight and bias of the hidden-node, and β is the output weight. In SVM, the latest LIBSVM software package 3.22 version is applied with the radial base function (RBF) as the kernel function. The regularization parameter C and the kernel width g are selected according to the grid search method. In both ELM and SVM, fifty trials have been conducted with training and testing datasets randomly generated for each trial, where the size of training and testing datasets is equal. All of the parameters in our experiments are summarized specifically in Table 2.

Firstly, we reveal the practicability of proposed feature KRF for discriminating seizure and non-seizure EEGs as shown in Figs. 5 and 6. Figure 5 demonstrates the kernel radius corresponding to a non-seizure and seizure EEG

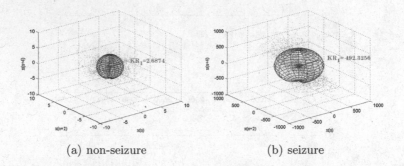

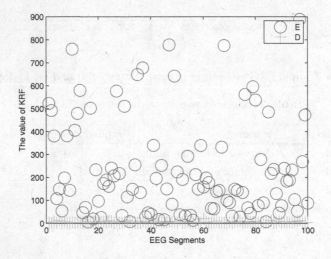

(a) non-seizure   (b) seizure

Fig. 5. The kernel radius corresponding to a non-seizure EEG and seizure EEG

Fig. 6. The values of KRF corresponding to EEG segments of set D and set E

respectively. It is obvious that the kernel radius 2.6874 corresponding to non-seizure EEG is much smaller than the kernel radius 492.3256 corresponding to seizure EEG, which shows that the proposed feature KRF is able to differentiate seizure EEGs and non-seizure EEGs successfully. Such fact can also been illustrated in Fig. 6.

Next, a comparative study between ELM and SVM is done with the same feature KRF. Experiments results are shown in Table 3, which include accuracy, standard deviation of accuracy and training time. We can observe from Table 3 that the classification accuracy obtained by ELM is a little better than that obtained by SVM with much smaller standard variation. It means that a better and stabler performance of epileptic seizure detection can be achieved by using KRF and ELM. Meanwhile, ELM spends much less time than SVM.

Finally, we compare the proposed automated seizure detection method KRF-ELM with other existing methods where the same datasets (i.e., D and E) are applied in simulations. We can observe from Table 4 that the proposed method

Table 3. Performance comparison between ELM and SVM with the same feature KRF

Classifier	Time	Accuracy	Standard deviation
ELM	0.0022	96.64%	0.0180
SVM	7.93	96.00%	3.1

Table 4. A comparison between the proposed methods in this paper and the methodologies in other literatures

Authors	Year	Methods	$CA(\%)$
Qi yuan et al. [19]	2012	Approximate entropy+ELM	$88.00 \pm 0.75\%$
	2012	Hurst exponent+ELM	$88.00 \pm 0.5\%$
	2012	DFA+ELM	$82.00 \pm 0.5\%$
Nicolaou et al. [11]	2012	Permutation entropy+SVM	83.13%
Zhu et al. [21]	2014	Degree and Strength of HVG+KNN	93%
Siuly et al. [14]	2011	Clustering+SVM	93.6%
Y. Kumar et al. [7]	2014	Fuzzy approximate entropy+SVM	95.85%
J.-L. Song et al. [15]	2016	lagged-$Poinca\acute{r}e$ based feature+ELM	96.16%
This paper		KRF+ELM	96.64%

KRF-ELM performs better than others. Even for the best and the most recent results obtained in [15], the classification accuracy obtained by our method increases from 96.16% to 96.64%.

4   Conclusion

In this work, we proposed the kernel-radius-based feature extraction method, where the kernel radius of three-dimensional phase space representation (3D-PSR) of intrinsic mode functions (IMFs) is defined to be the feature, which is further applied to differentiate seizure EEGs from non-seizure EEGs in accordance with the following procedures. At the first step, the given EEG signal is decomposed into different numbers of intrinsic mode functions (IMFs) adaptively by empirical mode decomposition (EMD) method; At the second step, the 3D-PSR is reconstructed for each IMF according to the time delay method; At the third step, the kernel radius of the corresponding 3D-PSR is defined, which aims to characterize the concentration degree of all the points in 3D-PSR. Combining with ELM and SVM, performances of the proposed method are finally verified on the open EEG database from three aspects: (1) performance verification of the proposed feature KRF; (2) performance comparison between ELM and SVM with the same feature KRF; (3) performance comparison between the proposed seizure detection method KRF-ELM with other existing methods. All the experimental results have demonstrated that the proposed method does a good job in the automated seizure detection.

Acknowledgement. This work was supported by the National Natural Science Foundation of China under Grant 61473223.

References

1. Acharya, U.R., Molinari, F., Subbhuraam, V.S., Chattopadhyay, S.: Automated diagnosis of epileptic EEG using entropies. Biomed. Signal Process. Control **7**, 401–408 (2012)
2. Chen, L.L., Zhang, J., Zou, J.Z., Zhao, C.J., Wang, G.S.: A frame work on wavelet-based nonlinear features and extreme learning machine for epileptic seizure detection. Biomed. Signal Process. Control **10**, 1–10 (2014)
3. Correa, A.G., Orosco, L., Diez, P., Laciar, E.: Automatic detection of epileptic seizures in longterm EEG records. Comput. Biol. Med. **57**, 66–73 (2015)
4. Takens, F.: Detecting strange attractors in turbulence. In: Rand, D., Young, L.-S. (eds.) Dynamical Systems and Turbulence, Warwick 1980. LNM, vol. 898, pp. 366–381. Springer, Heidelberg (1981). doi:10.1007/BFb0091924
5. Huang, N.E., Zheng, S., Long, S.R., Wu, M.C.: The empirical mode decomposition and the hilbert spectrum for nonlinear and non-stationary time series analysis. Proc. R. Soc. London Ser. A Math. Phys. Eng. Sci. **454**, 903–995 (1998)
6. Song, J.-L., Zhang, R.: Automated detection of epileptic EEGS using a novel fusion feature and extreme learning machine. Neurocomputing **175**, 383–391 (2016)
7. Kumar, Y., Dewal, M.L., Anand, R.S.: Epileptic seizuredetection using DWT based fuzzy approximate entropy and support vector machine. Neurocomputing **133**, 271–279 (2014)
8. Li, S.F., Zhong, W.D., Yuan, Q., Geng, S.J., Cai, D.M.: Feature extraction and recognition of ictal EEG using EMD and SVM. Comput. Biol. Med. **43**, 807–816 (2013)
9. Niknazar, M., Mousavi, S.R.: A new dissimilarity index of EEG signals for epileptic seizure detection. In: Control and Signal Processing, pp. 1–5 (2010)
10. Niknazar, M., Mousavi, S.R., Shamsollahi, M., Vahdat, B.V., Sayyah, M., Motaghi, S., Dehghani, A., Noorbakhsh, S.: Application of a dissimilarity index of EEG and its sub-bands on prediction of induced epileptic seizures from rat's EEG signals. IRBM **33**, 298–307 (2012)
11. Nicolaou, N., Georgiou, J.: Detection of epileptic electroencephalogram based on permutation entropy and support vector machines. Expert Syst. Appl. **39**, 202–209 (2012)
12. Ouyang, G., Li, X.L., Guan, X.P.: Use of fuzzy similarity index for epileptic seizure prediction. In: The 5th World Congress on Intelligent Control and Automation, Hang Zhou, China, vol. 6, pp. 5351–5355 (2004)
13. Quyen, M.L.V., Mattinerie, J., Navarro, V., Boon, P., DHave, M., Adam, C.: Anticipation of epileptic seizures from standard EEG recordings. Lancer **357**, 183–188 (2001)
14. Siuly, Y., Wen, P.P.: Clustering technique-based least square support vector machine for EEG signal classification. Comput. Meth. Prog. Biomed **104**, 358–372 (2011)
15. Song, J.L., Zhang, R.: Application of extreme learning machine to epileptic seizure detection based on lagged poincare plots. Multidimension. Syst. Signal Process. **28**, 945–959 (2017)

16. Song, Y., Crowcroft, J., Zhang, J.: Automated epileptic seizure detection in EEGs based on optimized sample entropy and extreme learning machine. J. Neurosci. Methods **210**, 132–146 (2012)
17. Tito, M., Cabrerizo, M., Ayala, M., Barreto, A., Miller, I., Jayakar, P., Adjouadi, M.: Classification of electroencephalographic seizure recordings into ictal and inter-ictal files using correlation sum. Comput. Biol. Med. **39**, 604–614 (2009)
18. Übeylia, E.D., Güler, I.: Detection of electrocardiographic changes in partial epilep-tic patients using lyapunov exponents with multilayer perceptron neural networks. Eng. Appl. Artif. Intell. **17**, 567–576 (2004)
19. Yuan, Q., Zhou, W., Li, S., Cai, D.: Epileptic EEG classification based on extreme learning machine and nonlinear features. Epilepsy Res. **96**, 29–38 (2011)
20. Zhang, Y.L., Zhou, W.D., Yuan, S.S., Yuan, Q.: Seizure detection method based on fractal dimension and gradient boosting. Epilepsy Behav. **43**, 30–38 (2015)
21. Zhu, G., Li, Y., Wen, P.: Epileptic seizure detection in eegs signals using a fast weighted horizontal visibility algorithm. Comput. Biol. Med. **115**, 64–75 (2014)

Some Directions of Medical Informatics in Russia

Nikita Shklovskiy-Kordi[1(✉)] (iD), Michael Shifrin[2], Boris Zingerman[1],
and Andrei Vorobiev[1]

[1] National Research Center for Hematology, Moscow, Russian Federation
nikitashk@gmail.com
[2] Burdenko's Neurosurgical Centre, Moscow, Russian Federation
shifrin@nsi.ru

Abstract. Israel Gelfand, one of the leaders of 20th century mathematics, devoted many years to biology and medical informatics. The directions, created by him, are not well known, but the main ideas are relevant even now. The ideology of the medical knowledge formalization was applied in developing by Michael Shifrin in Medical Information System of the Burdenko's Neurosurgery Institute. Under directorship of Andrei Vorobiev (Gelfand's disciple-physician), one of the largest healthcare informatizations of the 20th century was done: unified system introduced in most blood banks of the Russian Federation. Accompanying, obtaining, storing and distributing blood products "from the donor's vein to the patient's vein", the National Standard for Labeling Blood Products and the Law on Donation (with the task of forming the Unified Transfusion Information Space) were done. The same team, led by mathematician Boris Zingerman, developed the Medical Information System of the National Research Hematology Center, which was conceived as a unified system for managing all functions of the institution (out-patients and in-patients clinics, blood bank, pharmacy, research, accounting, personnel department and administration). The system focused on the full electronic document circulation with a single identification of participants and objects (including information objects). The National Standard "Electronic Case History" was created with the concepts of the Electronic Medical Record (EMR) first formulated as well as a number of other important definitions. The ideology of "Disease Image", based on the graphic presentation of data and the presentation of all medical events (records) from the EMR on a single time axis became the realization of Gelfand's idea of using physician experience for generation of intellectual algorithms in medical informatics.

Keywords: Patient health records (PHR) · Electronic Medical Record (EMR) · Integral medical data presentation · Intellectual algorithms · Distant medical monitoring

1 Gelfand's Approach to Medical Informatics

Modern "E-medicine" stands on three pillars: electronic document management, formalized plan of the medical history and the allocation of intellectual algorithms from medical thinking. Israel Gelfand began his research in the field of medical informatics in the late 1960s, when this term was not used yet. At that time, it was about applying

© Springer International Publishing AG 2017
S. Siuly et al. (Eds.): HIS 2017, LNCS 10594, pp. 22–31, 2017.
https://doi.org/10.1007/978-3-319-69182-4_3

the idea of pattern recognition to the tasks of medical diagnosis and forecasting. Ideologically and technically, Gelfand's approach was based on the work of Michael Bongard and his colleagues [1].

Already the first works in this direction (see details in [2]) led to three basic requirements for the future approach:

1.1 the results should be useful to the doctor for making decisions regarding the treatment of the particular patient;
1.2 methods of analysis should use the knowledge and experience of clinicians;
1.3 the results should be as conclusive as the results of experiments in biology and psychology.

The implementation of these provisions led to the central concept of adequate formalization and structuring of data, and to the method of diagnostic games – an instrument for identifying and formalizing expert knowledge. Later [3], these ideas were supplemented by an analysis of the early stages of work, in which the physician's desire to analyze the way to improve the treatment of his patients turns into a clearly stated formal task. As a result, a holistic approach to the use of formal methods in clinical medicine was developed, covering all stages of joint work of mathematicians and doctors, from the initial setting of the problem to the introduction of results into medical practice.

The needs for efficient organization of national system of Blood banks, complex diagnostic and verification of diagnosis from other hospitals brings doctor Vorobiev's team to computerization of clinical routine in 80-is. Require reference to primary diagnostic data, such as morphological images, analysis of disease progression and treatment outcome in their temporary occurrence and causal connections inspires creation of informatics instrument for management of clinical data. The following principles implemented:

- The system should be patient-focused. This led us to a common time-axis design rather than hierarchical structure for data analysis.
- The system should permit easy communications between health providers of different specialties. Thus, it has to accommodate different documents, such as text files, pictures, laboratory results, and others.
- To make it appealing for a wide range of users, the system has to be user-friendly and cost effective.

1.1 Personal Applicability of the Result

When doctor makes the decision about the treatment at the patient's bed, he must take into account a huge number of factors. But when the doctor is engaged in scientific work, he analyzes a limited set of data about a group of patients, and the individuality of patients is erased. A logical question arises: how to conduct a scientific analysis so that its results are adequate to the needs of the clinic and are useful for making decisions concerning specific patients?

In the course of the work, the frequently used notion of "clinical research" was clarified: it is "a work in which a question that makes sense for one patient is posed, and the main tool for its solution is the analysis of clinical data on a group of patients." On the basis of this concept, a chain "the medical goal - the adoption of a medical decision - the question of the patient - the task" was proposed (see [3]).

The medical goal forms a context in which the solution of the formal problem will be evaluated. The analysis of the decisions made by the doctor during the treatment of the patient makes it possible to identify the decisions that are of the greatest importance for achieving the stated goal. At the same time, we are looking for that specific question about the patient, the knowledge of the answer to which is important for making a decision about treatment, and which lends itself to formalization in the form of a task. At this stage of work, poorly formalized questions like "Does the patient have an operation?" Or "Which treatment is best?" are transformed into questions that are more amenable to formal analysis such as "Does the patient feel threatened by a relapse of the condition that led him to the clinic?" or "What is the prognosis of the outcome of treatment when using a particular method?".

1.2   Using the Experience of a Doctor

The need-for decision-making, regardless of availability of sufficient information at the moment is one of the essential features of the doctor's work. On the other hand, the doctor almost always has an excess of information about the patient, and he must isolate and discard those factors that in this particular case are not needed to make a decision. And it is the amazing ability of a person to make right decisions in a situation where information is both small and too much, allows him to solve problems that are inaccessible to formal methods of analysis. How to use this unique skill, which finds a concentrated expression in the experience and intuition of the doctor, for setting and solving formal problems?

Fundamental role in the described approach was played by the hypothesis about the structural organization of data by a person: for decision making, a person uses a small number of integral concepts - structural units - organizing the description of the objects in question in accordance with knowledge, experience and, very significantly, the objectives of the activity. One of the sources of this hypothesis was the biological work of Israel Gelfand (see [4]). But how to discover and describe these structural units, which can be regarded as the quintessence of professional experience, but which, more often than not, are formed implicitly?

Of course, in almost all works in which formal methods are used to solve medical problems, medical experience is used to some extent. But on the way to its identification and formalization, there is a significant obstacle. Everybody knows how difficult is to explain "intuition" decision made. Treating a patient and transferring his experience to students or to other doctors are two different activities. The experience of the doctor finds his immediate, but implicit expression at the patient's bedside, when the doctor's goal is to help a particular person. When a doctor looks for an explicit expression of his experience and builds an explanation of his actions, he pursues other goals, of a scientific or pedagogical nature, and often involuntarily introduces distortions into his description.

Even more difficult is the situation with the formalization of experience, because it requires a different, different from the medical culture of thinking. Let us emphasize that this culture of thinking, which is, conditionally speaking, "mathematicians", is not better or worse than the medical one, it is simply different, and the approach created by Israel Gelfand makes it possible to combine these two cultures in joint work for effective acquisition of new knowledge.

Since the best experience of the doctor is manifested in solving practical problems, a special experimental method was developed to identify the medical experience - "diagnostic games" - when using which the doctor answers natural questions for him, such as diagnosis and prognosis of the course of the disease. The peculiarity of this technique, close to the psychological experiment, is that the physician takes a natural decision for him, being in a controlled information environment: he receives all the necessary data about the patient in strictly "metered" volume from other participants in the work. Thus, during diagnostic games the doctor solves problems that are close to those he decides every day, and at the same time, it is precisely known what data about the patient he uses to solve them.

1.3   Proof of the Result

Reliability and reproducibility of the results are the most important conditions for their applicability. To achieve this, a number of techniques similar to those used in biology, psychology, and clinical trials have been developed. These include:

- Requirements for the formulation of the problem, including, the exact wording of the question, the criteria for verifying the answers, an accurate description of the contingent of patients for whom the problem is being solved, and the initial data used in the analysis;
- Requirements for the preparation of formalized information cards;
- a detailed description of the technique of diagnostic games, which avoids the implicit use of data; In particular, techniques similar to the double-blind method are used, · which allow to avoid implicit prompts and bias of the doctor's answers;
- The mandatory stage of the "clinical verification" of the result, when the formal solution of the problem is applied to the current contingent of patients, but the answer is not reported to the doctor, and much more. In the book [2] a great attention has been paid to these questions.

It is worth paying attention to the great importance attached to setting the problem and collecting the initial data for formal analysis. Negligence in any of these cases can negate the results of the most sophisticated methods of analysis.

The main idea of Gelfand's approach to medical informatics can be expressed very briefly: "medical informatics is the formalization of the doctor's activity". This formulation has two interesting features (for details, see [5]):

- It does not exhaust medical informatics - and cannot claim it, like any other wording relating to such a complex subject;

- It is simple, but its disclosure is difficult, requires the development of a special language and special methods to implement it and obtain real results.

As a consequence of this complexity, these theses left behind many important aspects of Gelfand's approach to the problems of medical informatics. One of the most impressive is the ability to work effectively with small samples typical of clinical medicine. Using structural units allows you to work in a situation where the number of signs used to describe the state of patients is an order of magnitude greater than the number of cases available for analysis. Structural organization of data makes it possible to rely on existing links between characteristics in contrast to many statistical methods of analysis that require the independence of signs. Surprisingly, in very difficult medical issues, it was possible to find a small - 5–7 - number of structural units, in terms of which the problem was solved. Due to various reasons, Gelfand's approach to medical informatics has not been widely used, although some of his elements can be found in so many works. It is to be hoped that the recent publications of the author and his colleagues (see [6, 7]) popularize this approach and give impetus to its development under the new conditions. Internet, instant communications, globally distributed information systems and databases, etc. - all this creates a fundamentally new information environment in which collective human activity is taking place - but does not in the least reduce the importance of individual professional skill. Moreover, an adequately formalized expert experience can be disseminated and analyzed much more quickly and deeper than before.

2   Medical Information System "Transfusiology"

The team of information system developers formed on the basis of the National Research Center for Hematology implements set of projects in the field of transfusiology:

- The project of the Automated Blood Transfusion Information Station (1989), introduced in various configurations in more than 30 Blood Bunks and hospitals in Russia and the Former Soviet Union;
- Priority development and implementation of the barcode labeling and identification system in transfusiology;
- 30 years (up to the present) of development, operation, adaptation to new regulatory requirements, and the expansion of the functional of the Transfusiology Information System of the National Research Center for Hematology;
- Independent development and constant participation in the development of key regulatory documents regulating the use of IT in transfusiology:
  - Technical regulations,
  - Industry classifier of blood components
  - Draft National Standard "Components of blood. Classification"
  - Specialized classifiers for the National Blood Service project
  - The first and so far the only National Standard in the field of Transfusiology GOST R 52938-2008 "Donor blood and its components. Containers with preserved blood or its components. Marking."
- Production of blood components:

- Registration and withdrawal of donors, maintenance of donor and tape files
- Interaction with donors through an external portal (recording for donation, informing, SMS reminders calls for donation and re-examination, congratulations, thank you letters, "honor board")
- Donor screening, referral to donation
- Preparation of donation (blood lead or apheresis) and recording of its results
- Production of blood components (fractionation)
- Laboratory testing of blood components, culling
- Marking of blood components
- Quarantine of plasma
- Viral infection of blood components
- Freezing, defrosting of blood cells, long-term storage bank
- Storage, reception of external products, selection, optimization and issuance at the request of offices
- Reporting
- Investigations, analytics, statistical processing [8].

The concept of creation and functioning of the Automated Information System of Clinical Transfusiology, integrated both with the Automated Information System of Transfusiology (production, blood service) - and with the State Health Information System is formulated. Solutions are proposed for ensuring transparency not only in obtaining donor blood components, but also in their clinical application. The introduction of information systems into the practice of not only the blood service institutions, but also other medical organizations, is aimed at raising the level of safety, obtaining on-line objective and reliable data on the efficacy of transfusion and transfusion complications, and keeping a constant record-keeping and monitoring. Specialized information modules included in the Unified Information Space of Transfusiology allow forming communication with donors through social networks. A system for informing donors about the use of blood components handed over to them for therapeutic purposes is being tested. Modules and algorithms for downloading information about the state of health of the donor successfully work. Information received in the process of preparing for donation of blood components (medical examination of the donor) and information obtained during processing and testing of blood products, is loaded into the Personal Electronic Medical Card of the donor. The medical card is linked to mobile applications for donors, offering information materials and a donor calendar. Thus, a system of donor involvement in the care of one's own health is formed.

3 Time-Oriented Multi-image Case History – Way to the "Disease Image" Analysis

Under directorship of Andrei Vorobiov (Gelfand's disciple-physician) team led by mathematician Boris Zingerman developed the Medical Information System for the National Hematology Center, which was conceived as a unified system for managing all functions of the institution (clinic, blood bank, pharmacy, accounting, personnel department and other administration). The system was focused on the full electronic document circulation with a single identification of participants and objects (including information objects). The National Standard "Electronic Case History" was created with the concepts of the Electronic Medical Record (EMR) first formulated. The ideology of "disease image", based on the graphic integration of the EMR and the presentation of all medical events on a single time axis was developed.

An example of Intellectual algorithm born inside medical process is the logical structuring of data known as "temperature sheets" where leading parameters and therapeutic assignments on one sheet of observation have a common time axis. This algorithm has helped to develop the system of biological dosimetry – the core element of the acute irradiation disease, as well as protocols for treatment of acute leukemia and other hematologic malignancies [9]. We used the following steps in preforming this intellectual algorithm in computer program:

1. Integration of data stored in different formats (text, tables, roentgenograms, microphotographs, videos etc.);
2. Compression of clinical data by highlighting important and urgent information;
3. Display of information in an integrated fashion on the same screen;
4. Automatic matching of entered data with stored timetables derived from established protocols for diagnostic procedures and treatment.
5. Generation of warning signs ("flags") wherever the data indicate divergence from specified protocols. Exit from the assigned limits of selected parameters is similarly controlled. When a standard protocol is used for management of a patient with defined diagnosis, a template is provided with required laboratory data and medications to be used with a timetable for their administration.

Therapy: The appropriate medication is selected from a list provided for the individual patient according to diagnosis. If a particular medication is absent from the list, it can be entered using the pharmacological reference database online. Drugs on each line can be selected by cursor for each day followed by pressing a button "therapy" which enters the dose for each specific medication.

Events.   Significant events and diagnostic procedures are recorded by selection from a common list or by entering a descriptive term. The user marks the significance of each event by color coding and enters information on the given event. Files representing morphological images, roentgenogram, text documents, etc. can be attached to a specific time period by the indicating of the file's address. After filling the "event form", a cursor tags the event to a "window" for a brief description. A double click opens a map of all pictures and text files linked to the event.

Laboratory data.   All test results for a particular patient for each specific time are entered in this appropriate field.

Normalization.   All numeric clinical data is broken into normal, sub-normal and pathological range with values stored. This provides normalization of all parameters and presentation by using common axes. Division of the measured value by the accepted average value accomplishes the normalization. The calculation is executed separately for normal, sub-normal and pathological values. To define the range of sub-normal values, a team of experts empirically established the scope of "acceptable" (for the given diagnosis and selected method of therapy and, in some cases, for an individual patient) parameters. If a parameter stays within the defined sub-normal or normal range, no special action is required. The pathological range covers all the zone of possible values beyond the sub-normal values. In case of manual input, under the date of the analysis, the measured value should be entered. The cell on is automatically converted to the color conforming its position on a scale of normal or pathologic range. If the specific value is out of the acceptance limits, the program generates an automatic alarm signal.

Complications. Complications are recorded on a specific line and serves for visualization of the dynamics of patient's symptoms. After a symptom/syndrome is selected from a pre-loaded list, a window appears on the screen with a definition and criteria to assist in the diagnosis and management. Additional functions are available for further user assistance.

The standard format for presenting key components of patient's medical record (the constant form of a positional relationship of the basic semantic units of a case history) was developed. It has the flexibility for adding templates, as necessary for a specific diagnosis. These templates accumulate pre-defined lists of medications, lab tests and syndromes, and define range of values for normalization, as well as color palette. Also,

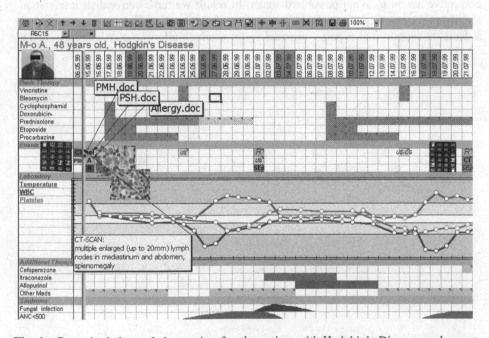

Fig. 1. Comprised sheet of observation for the patient with Hodgkin's Disease, underwent chemotherapy. Some information presented as marks only, some as small windows. The dynamics of chosen parameters (Temperature, WBC and Platelet counts) are normalized and color-coded. (Color figure online)

the template may refer to the standard protocols for specific diseases or clinical trials stored in the database [10–13] (Fig. 1).

The beforehand constructed template permits standard recognized images for diagnosis and helps to discriminate general characteristics and specific features for an individual patient. For example, there are accepted criteria for decrease in platelets, leukocyte and hemoglobin in response to chemotherapeutic treatment. Slower recovery indicates a poor bone marrow reserve, severe infection or other complications. We found that comparison of shapes of drug-dependent changes in blood counts is a valuable estimation of outcome.

In a real-time mode, the system automatically performed data validation and notified a user when selected parameters were beyond acceptable ranges or when the timetable set by the protocol was not followed. These software features permit health care personnel to monitor and correct, when needed, individual actions taken by medical personnel. The system links the actions of medical staff with requirements set by the protocols, thus minimizing the potential risk of complications. Attention of physicians and staff is prompted by a color indicator, which signals "inquiries - interlocks". Depending on the type of error, the system suggests several responses. These include cancellation of an inquiry or change in assigned medication or dosage. Notification of specific violation is automatically dispatched to the address of the individual in charge of the protocol management, primary physician or other personnel specified by the user. Thus, the error is detected in real-time and the system facilitates collective decisions for corrective action to avoid possible damage. In result we have convenient intellectual algorithm for entering all available information about a patient. It may be classified as a decision-support and expert – oriented system, which allows a physician to select a

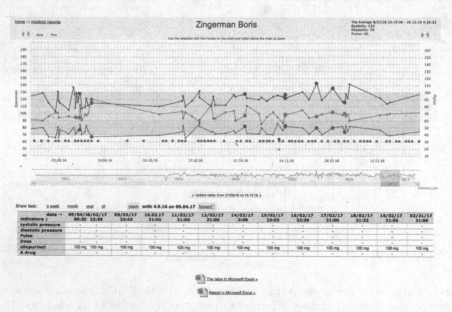

Fig. 2. Scalable representation mobile application self-monitoring blood pressure and pulse on WWW.MEDARHIV.RU.

pre-entered template and to modify it for creating the most appropriate template for a particular patient. It provides easy access to primary data and allows generation of a common time-line axis format for multimedia presentation of a patient's record. The system links multi-format medical data forming a recognizable image of disease, allows its real-time evaluation. Today graphical integration of medical data can be represented as scalable single time axe multimedia Internet-based instruments (Fig. 2).

Acknowledgements. This work was supported, in part, by a Grants RFBR, Russia № 16-29-12998, № 16-07-01140, № 16-07-01047.

References

1. Bongard, M.M.: The problem of recognition (Russ.). "Nauka" Publication, Moscow (1967)
2. Gelfand, I.M., Rosenfeld, B.I., Shifrin, M.A.: Essays on the joint work of mathematicians and doctors (Russ.). "Nauka" Publication, Moscow (2005)
3. Alekseevsky, A.V., Gelfand, I.M., Izvekova, M.L., Shifrin, M.A.: On the Role of Formal Methods in the Clinical: From the Goal to the Formulation of the Problem (Russ.). "Nauka" Publication, Moscow (1997)
4. Vasiliev, Y.M., Gelfand, I.M., Guberman, S.A., Shik, M.L.: Interaction in biological systems (Russ.). Nauka **6**, 7 (1969)
5. Shifrin, M.A.: On the Simple and Complex in Informatics - News of Artificial Intelligence, N 2 (2005)
6. Shifrin, M.A., Belousova O.B., Kasparova E.I.: Diagnostic games, a tool for clinical experience formalization in interactive "Physician-IT-specialist" framework. In: Proceedings of the Twentieth IEEE International Symposium on Computer-Based Medical Systems (2007)
7. Shifrin, M.A., Kasparova, E.I.: Diagnostic games: from adequate formalization of clinical experience to structure discovery. In: Proceedings of the 21st European Congress of Medical Informatics, pp. 57–62 (2008)
8. Zingerman, B., Kobelyatsky, V., Gorodetskiy, V.: Information technology in transfusiology and the task of creating a Unified Information Space (Russ.). Hematol. Transfusiology **51**(3), 36–41 (2007)
9. Vorobiev, A.I., Brilliant, M.D.: WBC and Platelets dynamic during acute irradiation syndrome as biological dosimeter (Russ.) In: Proceeding of Conference in Institute of Biophysics, Moscow (1970)
10. Shklovskiy-Kordi, N., Zingerman, B., et al.: A time axis Presentation of the clinical and diagnostic information from multiple sources. J. Am. Assoc. Med. Inform. Supplement, 1161 (1999)
11. Shklovskiy-Kordi, N., Freidin, J., et al.: Standardization for telemedical consultation on a basis of multimedia case history. In: Proceedings, Fourteenth IEEE Symposium on Computer-Based Medical Systems, pp. 535–540 (2001)
12. Goldberg, S., Shklovskiy-Kordi, N., Zingerman, B.: Time-oriented multi-image case history - the way to the "disease image analysis". In: VISAPP, Barcelona, Spain, pp. 378–383 (2007)
13. Shklovskiy-Kordi, N., Zingerman, B., Varticovski, L.: Electronic Health Records (EHR) adapted for clinical trials. J. Clin. Oncol. **29**(15_suppl), 345–346 (2011)

A Computer Simulation Approach to Reduce Appointment Lead-Time in Outpatient Perinatology Departments: A Case Study in a Maternal-Child Hospital

Miguel Ortíz-Barrios[1(✉)], Genett Jimenez-Delgado[2],
and Jeferson De Avila-Villalobos[1]

[1] Department of Industrial Management, Agroindustry and Operations,
Universidad de la Costa CUC, Barranquilla, Colombia
{mortiz1,jdeavila8}@cuc.edu.co
[2] Department of Industrial Processes Engineering, Institución Universitaria ITSA,
Soledad, Colombia
gjimenez@itsa.edu.co

Abstract. A significant problem in outpatient perinatology departments is the long waiting time for pregnant women to receive an appointment. In this respect, appointment delays are related to patient dissatisfaction, no shows and sudden infant death syndrome. This paper aims to model and evaluate improvement proposals to outpatient care delivery by applying computer simulation approaches. First, suitable data is collected and analyzed. Then, a discrete-event simulation (DES) model is created and validated to determine whether it is statistically equivalent to the current system. Afterward, the average appointment lead-time is calculated and studied. Finally, improvement proposals are designed and pretested by simulation modelling and statistical comparison tests. A case study of an outpatient perinatology department from a maternal-child is shown to validate the effectiveness of DES to fully understand and manage healthcare systems. The results evidenced that changes to care delivery can be effectively assessed and appointment lead-times may be significantly reduced based on the proposed framework within this paper.

Keywords: Discrete-event simulation (DES) · Perinatology · Outpatient care appointment lead-time · Healthcare

1 Introduction

Outpatient perinatology departments have been facing increased demands in emerging countries while addressing financial difficulties limiting the implementation of improvements to care delivery. This has resulted in longer appointment lead-times which could become a significant problem in the future as demands on outpatient perinatology services continue to rise [1]. Delayed appointments can have a detrimental effect on attendance rates [2] and patient satisfaction levels [3]. Additionally, long lead times are associated with delayed diagnosis and treatment which contributes to the use of more complex healthcare services (e.g. hospitalization, emergency and intensive care),

S. Siuly et al. (Eds.): HIS 2017, LNCS 10594, pp. 32–39, 2017.
https://doi.org/10.1007/978-3-319-69182-4_4

development of more severe complications in pregnant women and the increase of fetal, infant and maternal mortality indexes [4]. This is even more important since the perinatology appointments are assigned to women with a high-risk pregnancy. In this regard, the appointment lead-time is a pivotal parameter that should now be addressed to increase the response of outpatient perinatology departments to patients.

To provide an efficient solution to this problem, discrete event simulation (DES) has been widely used to underpin the decision-making process derived from this increasing need [5]. In this regard, DES ensures modelling the throughput of outpatient departments which enables decision makers to fully understand the internal interactions by using suitable data [6]. However, in spite of the extensive reported literature related to the use of DES in healthcare services, a review developed by [5] reveals that this technique has been poorly applied when pretesting changes to care delivery and the evidence base is very small.

In an effort to address this problem and cover the literature gap, in this paper we model the outpatient perinatology department of a maternal-child hospital, initially with the purpose of establishing a baseline compared to three improvement scenarios could be assessed. The novelty of this work lies in the use of DES to minimizing appointment lead-times in a perinatology department which has not been reported in the literature. Furthermore, after validation, improvement scenarios can be pretested before implementation. Therefore, this research will provide a safe and efficient guideline for both healthcare managers and practitioners and consequently, a significant offering for society.

The remainder of this paper is organized as follows: in Sect. 2, a brief literature review relating to improvement strategies for outpatient perinatology departments is presented; Sect. 3 describes and analyzes the results of a case study from a maternal-child hospital. Finally, Sect. 4 presents the conclusions and future work emanating from this study.

2 Related Work

The Discrete Event Simulation (DES) is a technique creating models based on equipment and software [22]. This helps to analyze the system performance under different conditions by pretesting possible changes and their effects [7, 8]. However, the benefits of simulation approaches in decision making (e.g. cost savings, process optimization and increased customer satisfaction) are not yet fully extended in organizations, including those from the healthcare sector. In this regard, the scientific literature reports studies on the application of DES aiming at characterizing, evaluating alternatives and improving operations.

In this respect, we found scientific articles that demonstrate the use of DES techniques to underpin the improvement in the delivery of ambulatory health services [9]. There is also evidence related to use of DES approaches as a managerial support tool for the improvement of specific healthcare services: physiotherapy [10], gynecology and obstetrics [3], internal medicine [11], mammography [12], outpatient specialties [13], stroke care units [14] and radiotherapy [15]. Additionally, the simulation helps to model healthcare processes from an integral perspective and can be also combined with different methodologies, e.g. lean design [16], queuing theory [17], mathematical optimization models [18] and system dynamics [19]. We also found studies with DES applications implemented for the design and configuration of health centers [20, 21]. Particularly, this research focuses on the use of the DES techniques to minimize waiting times in outpatient perinatology departments. In this respect, very few studies were found in the scientific literature. In [3], the authors presented a DES application where appointment lead-time was reduced in a unit of gynecology and obstetrics. On the other hand, in [22], a DES technique was used as a teaching strategy for acquisition and retention of clinical skills to the delivery of neonatology services. This confirms the results exposed by [5] where it was concluded that "in spite of DES has been validated as an efficient tool to pretest changes to healthcare delivery, the evidence base is too small and poorly developed". Therefore, this research contributes to the scientific literature and provides an efficient solution to outpatient perinatology departments when reducing both waiting time and appointment lead-time.

3   Modeling the Perinatology Department: A Case Study in a Maternal-Child Hospital

A case study of an outpatient perinatology department from a maternal-child hospital has been explored. The model details the journey of pregnant women from arrival time to discharge. The patients are pregnant women between the ages of 15 and 45 years old. Our model was based on a 5-year prospective dataset provided by the Statistics Department and consisting of all patients admitted between 1 January 2012 and 31 December 2016 and operates 9 h per day. Then, an independence test was carried out to determine whether the variable *time between arrivals* was random. To support this assumption, a run test was performed with $\alpha = 0.01$. The outcomes demonstrated with p-value = 0.538 that this variable could be fitted to a probability distribution. Then, the *time between arrivals variable* was concluded to be modelled with an exponential distribution ($\beta = 2.72$ h). For the goodness-of-fit, the Kolmogorov-Smirnov test (p-value = 0) provided good support for the exponential assumption.

Out of the total admissions, 66.6% ask for a perinatology appointment personally and the rest by phone service. If personally, two schedulers are available from 8 am to 5 pm with service time fitted to NORM (3.70, 1.78) hours with p-value < 0.01. On the contrary, if attended by phone, one scheduler is assigned with the same service time. As a result, the appointment is allocated to the patient according to the available time slots of doctors. In this respect, medical care is in charge of one doctor (perinatologist) whose service time can be modelled by a uniform probability distribution UNIF (1.05, 1.5) hours (p-value < 0.01). The opening hours for outpatient perinatology consultation are Thursdays mornings (8 am–12 pm) and Fridays (8 am–5 pm). Additionally, it is good to highlight that, on consultation day, the patients must firstly go to the billing department where two servers are available with service times fitted to uniform distribution UNIF (2.36, 5.72) minutes.

Outpatient perinatology departments are regulated by the Ministry of Health and Social Protection. In this regard, the upper specification limit (USL) for average appointment lead-time has been set as 8 min/admission. This information was considered in the simulation model that was created with the aid of Arena 14.5 ® software in order to minimize the current appointment lead-time of the perinatology department. A T-test was performed to determine whether the simulated model was statistically equivalent to the real system. In this respect, a P-value equal to 0.1812 and t = 1,359 evidenced that the model was statistically equal to the real-world system. Furthermore, the current average appointment lead-time was determined. On average, a pregnant woman has to wait for 6.36 days with a standard deviation of 1.45 days (refer to Fig. 1).

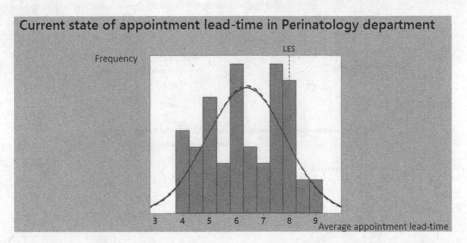

Fig. 1. Current performance of outpatient perinatology department in terms of average appointment lead-time

This represents a DPMO (Defects per million of opportunities) = 131067 which means that out of 1 million of admissions, 131067 will have to wait for more than 8 days before consultation date in perinatology department. In an effort to address this problem, three improvement proposals were created with the aid of hospital managers. Each proposal was pretested by using DES models before implementation (refer to Fig. 2a, b, c).

Proposal 1 suggests changing the perinatologist schedule. In this way, the doctor would work from Monday to Friday mornings (8 am–12 pm). On the other hand, Proposal 2 recommends adding one doctor with the current perinatologist schedule. Finally, Proposal 3 pretests implementing a set of two doctors: one with the current journey and the other with the schedule exposed in Proposal 1.

After evaluating these proposals, the performance indicators evidenced that all the proposals are satisfactory due to they provide a reduced appointment lead-time. In this respect, a T-test was performed to compare the current performance of the outpatient perinatology department and each improvement scenario. The results of these statistical analysis have been summarized in Table 1.

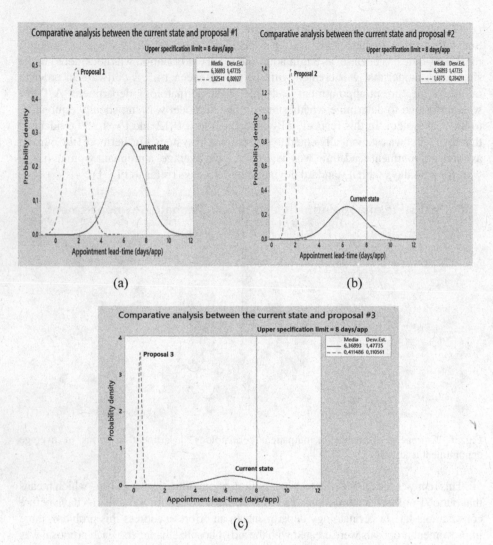

Fig. 2. Comparative analysis of current performance and Proposal 1 (a), Proposal 2 (b) and Proposal 3 (c)

Table 1. P-values, T statistics and confidence intervals for comparisons between real system and proposals

Proposal	P-value	T	CI for difference between means (95%)
Proposal 1	0	22.7	[4.140; 4.941]
Proposal 2	0	22.9	[4.320; 5.143]
Proposal 3	0	30.11	[5.561; 6.354]

Additionally, the improvement proposals were pairwise compared in terms of appointment lead-time via also performing T-tests (refer to Table 2). It can be concluded that the Proposal 3 provides the best operational performance due to its significant reduced variation. In addition, when combining the results from Tables 1 and 2, it can be fully appreciated that Proposal 3 offers an attractive solution for both hospital managers and pregnant women since it ensures an immediate access to perinatology consultation and care services are not overwhelmed in the long run. This would also contribute to reducing the rate of maternal mortality, healthcare costs and the development of pregnancy complications during pregnancy that may carry a high risk of severe fetal morbidity.

Table 2. P-values, T statistics and confidence intervals for comparisons between proposals

Pairwise comparison	P-value	T	CI for difference between means (95%)
Proposal 1–Proposal 2	0.007	2.88	[0.0566; 0.3250]
Proposal 1–Proposal 3	0	40.85	[1.3487; 1.4849]
Proposal 2–Proposal 3	0	20.63	[1.1036; 1.3484]

4   Conclusions and Future Work

In this paper, a discrete-event simulation approach was presented to reduce the average appointment lead-time in an outpatient perinatology department from a maternal-child hospital. During this application, it was proved that healthcare processes are very complex to model so it is, therefore, necessary to work closely with medical staff and healthcare managers to provide more realistic models. Whilst, the availability of suitable data is another aspect of concern to obtain a good representation of the real-world model. We thus need to incorporate high-quality data and information provided by the clinicians into the model.

Particularly, the results evidenced that considering the current outpatient perinatology department, pregnant women had to wait for 6.36 days with a standard deviation of 1.45 days before a consultation. Thus, three proposals were simulated and pretested with the support of Arena 14.5 ® software, Minitab 17 and conceptual aspects provided by the healthcare managers of the hospital. For this case study, all of the proposals were found to be operationally efficient since they offer a reduced appointment lead-time compared to the current department. However, the best proposal (Proposal 3) enable managers to minimize average appointment lead-time from 6.36 days to 3.7 h and the standard deviation from 1.47 days to 1 h. These outcomes are highly beneficial for pregnant women who will have a minor risk of sudden infant death syndrome and maternal mortality.

An additional aspect of interest to the healthcare managers is the possibility of pretesting changes to outpatient care delivery before implementation in an effective and safe manner by using computer simulation approach. The illustrative example presented in this paper enriches the reported literature since the evidence base is poorly developed. To this end, we plan in future work to implement cost models with the aim of fully supporting decision-making processes in healthcare institutions. Furthermore, our work will be extended towards considering other outpatient departments in order to validate the effectiveness of the proposed framework.

References

1. Giachetti, R.E.: A simulation study of interventions to reduce appointment lead-time and patient no-show rate. In: 2008 Winter Simulation Conference, pp. 1463–1468. IEEE (2008)
2. Canizares, M.J., Penneys, N.S.: The incidence of nonattendance at an urgent care dermatology clinic. J. Am. Acad. Dermatol. 46(3), 457–459 (2002)
3. Ortiz, M.A., McClean, S., Nugent, C.D., Castillo, A.: Reducing appointment lead-time in an outpatient department of gynecology and obstetrics through discrete-event simulation: a case study. In: García, C.R., Caballero-Gil, P., Burmester, M., Quesada-Arencibia, A. (eds.) UCAmI 2016. LNCS, vol. 10069, pp. 274–285. Springer, Cham (2016). doi: 10.1007/978-3-319-48746-5_28
4. Neal, R.D., Tharmanathan, P., France, B., Din, N.U., Cotton, S., Fallon-Ferguson, J., Hamilton, W., Hendry, A., Hendry, M., Lewis, R., Macleod, U., Mitchell, E.D., Pickett, M., Rai, T., Shaw, K., Stuart, N., Tørring, M.L., Wilkinson, C., Williams, B., Williams, N., Emery, J.: Is increased time to diagnosis and treatment in symptomatic cancer associated with poorer outcomes? Systematic review. Br. J. Cancer 112, S92–S107 (2015)
5. Mohiuddin, S., Busby, J., Savović, J., Richards, A., Northstone, K., Hollingworth, W., Donovan, J.L., Vasilakis, C.: Patient flow within UK emer-gency departments: a systematic review of the use of computer simulation modelling meth-ods. BMJ Open 7(5), e015007 (2017)
6. Gillespie, J., McClean, S., Garg, L., Barton, M., Scotney, B., Fullerton, K.: A multi-phase DES modelling framework for patient-centred care. J. Oper. Res. Soc. 67(10), 1239–1249 (2016)
7. Villanueva, J.: La Simulacion de Procesos, Clave en la Toma de Decisiones. Revista DYNA 83(4), 221–227 (2008)
8. Banks, J.: Introduction to simulation. In: Winter Simulation Conference, pp. 11–13 (1999)
9. Hong, T., Shang, P., Arumugam, M., Yusuff, R.: Use of simulation to solve outpatient clinic problems: A review of the literature. S. Afr. J. Ind. Eng. 24(3), 27–42 (2013)
10. Villamizar, J., Coelli, F., Pereira, W., Almeida, R.: Discrete-event computer simulation methods in the optimization of a physiotherapy clinic. Physiotherapy 97, 71–77 (2011)
11. Ortiz, M.A., López-Meza, P.: Using computer simulation to improve patient flow at an outpatient internal medicine department. In: García, C.R., Caballero-Gil, P., Burmester, M., Quesada-Arencibia, A. (eds.) UCAmI 2016. LNCS, vol. 10069, pp. 294–299. Springer, Cham (2016). doi:10.1007/978-3-319-48746-5_30
12. Coelli, F., Ferreira, R., Almeida, R., Pereira, W.: Computer simulation and discrete-event models in the analysis of a mammography clinic patient flow. Comput. Methods Programs Biomed. 87, 201–207 (2007)
13. Mocarzel, B., Shelton, D., Uyan, B., Pérez, E., Jimenez, J., DePagter, L.: Modeling and simulation of patient admission services in a multi-specialty outpatient clinic. In: Proceedings of the 2013 Winter Simulation Conference, pp. 2309–2319 (2013)
14. Pitt, M., Monks, T., Crowe, S., Vasilakis, C.: Systems modelling and simulation in health service design, delivery and decision making. BMJ Qual. Safety 25, 1–8 (2015)
15. Werker, G., Sauré, A., French, J., Shechter, S.: The use of discrete-event simulation modelling to improve radiation therapy planning processes. Radiother. Oncol. 92, 76–82 (2009)
16. Robinson, S., Radnorb, Z., Burgessc, N., Worthington, C.: SimLean: utilising simulation in the implementation of lean in healthcare. Eur. J. Oper. Res. 219, 188–197 (2012)
17. Bahadori, M., Mohammadnejhad, S., Ravangard, R., Teymourzadeh, E.: Using queuing theory and simulation model to optimize hospital pharmacy performance. Iran Red Crescent Med. J. 16(3), 1–7 (2014)

18. Granja, C., Almada-Lobo, B., Janela, F., Seabra, J., Mendes, A.: An optimization based on simulation approach to the patient admission scheduling problem using a linear programing algorithm. J. Biomed. Inform. **52**, 427–437 (2014)
19. Viana, J., Brailsford, S.C., Harindra, V., Harper, P.R.: Combining discrete-event simulation and system dynamics in a healthcare setting: A composite model for Chlamydia infection. Eur. J. Oper. Res. **237**, 196–206 (2014)
20. Swisher, J., Jacobson, S., Jun, B., Balci, O.: Modeling and analyzing a physician clinic environment using discrete-event (visual) simulation. Comput. Oper. Res. **28**, 105–125 (2001)
21. De Angelis, V., Felici, G., Impelluso, P.: Integrating simulation and optimization in health care centre management. Eur. J. Oper. Res. **150**, 101–114 (2003)
22. Herazo-Padilla, N., Montoya-Torres, J.R., Munoz-Villamizar, A., Nieto Isaza, S., Ramirez Polo, L.: Coupling ant colony optimization and discrete-event simulation to solve a stochastic location-routing problem. In: 2013 Simulations Conference (WSC), pp. 3352–3362. IEEE (2013)

Engaging Patients, Empowering Doctors in Digitalization of Healthcare

Nikita Shklovsky-Kordi[1]([✉]), Boris Zingerman[1], Michael Shifrin[2], Rostislav Borodin[3], Tatiana Shestakova[4], and Andrei Vorobiev[1]

[1] National Research Center for Hematology, Moscow, Russian Federation
nikitashk@gmail.com
[2] Burdenko's Neurosurgical Centre, Moscow, Russian Federation
shifrin@nsi.ru
[3] National Research University Higher School of Economics, Moscow, Russian Federation
roctbb@gmail.com
[4] Moscow Regional Research and Clinical Institute, Moscow, Russian Federation
t240169@yandex.ru

Abstract. Patients can monitor their own physiological parameters and medical events using mobile applications. The problem is how to involve patients in regular use. The key problem seems to convince the patient that doctor will get acquainted with the data sent in service of Patient Health Records (PHR) on time. From other hand we have to organize for doctors the comfortable access to such data and do not overload them. The dynamics of clinical parameters of diabetes, hypertension, anticoagulation – vital for successful treatment, so these patients and their physicians seems to be perspective for innovation methods. Pulse, blood pressure, weight, glucose level and confirmation of a dose of medication taken, organized to be immediately delivered in the PHR from mobile application and household measuring devices used by the patient. The doctor choosing variants of presentation of medical monitoring information transmitted from the patient. In addition, specialized Medical Messenger (MM) allows the patient to ask questions to the doctor at the moment when they arise without disturbing the life of the doctor via his personal mobile phone or e-mail. We expect this exchange of messages will serve as a base of innovative interactive case history, managed not only by physician, but by patient as well. Personal monitoring also used for evaluating the "adherence to treatment": system of reminders about medication and measurements, the results of which become available to doctor according intellectual algorithms he chooses.

Keywords: Patient health records (PHR) · Medical data presentation · Distant medical monitoring · Intellectual algorithms · Adherence to treatment

1 Introduction

Modern information and communication technologies provide unprecedented opportunities for involving patients in the treatment process, and all citizens - in the process of health management. But for the effective use of new technologies, one must not only

© Springer International Publishing AG 2017
S. Siuly et al. (Eds.): HIS 2017, LNCS 10594, pp. 40–44, 2017.
https://doi.org/10.1007/978-3-319-69182-4_5

entice new opportunities for patients, but also give the doctor tools for working in new conditions. And, above all, in conditions of remote communication with patients and increasing information flows. We will touch upon the tasks related to only one aspect of emerging digital health: remote monitoring of patient's condition.

The introduction of remote monitoring requires the solution of various tasks, of which the following are highlighted.

1. The patient should not spend much time inputting the results of his observations and measurements.
2. The patient should be sure that the doctor will see his data on time.
3. The doctor should be sure that he will not be bothered without proper grounds.
4. The physician must have effective tools for analyzing the incoming data.
5. The entire history of each patient's observations should be available to the physician.

The tools that are needed to solve these problems already exist, only a new look at them and integration is needed [1–3].

2 Methods and Discussion

The solution of these tasks is linked with the systems of personal medical records – PHR [4, 5]. The authors have experience in the design and use of the Patient Health Records (PHR) system WWW.MEDARHIV.RU, which has a number of rather specific properties [6]:

- Access rights to records are completely controlled by patients. In particular, the patient can allow his doctor to arrange consultations with other specialists.
- Each entry in the system can be accurately told whether it was made by the patient, by a doctor, or automatically came from some hospital information system [7–9]. This removes the frequently asked question about the degree of trust in records in the PHR class systems.
- The system is not associated with any particular medical institution or their network. Any institution can connect to it, if it is necessary for at least one patient.

The usual ways of communicating a patient with a doctor using a mobile phone, public messengers and e-mails have a number of significant drawbacks [10]. Patients can disturb the doctor - and this is actually observed, and often unambiguous identification of the patient is a big problem. The doctor, for his part, is overwhelmed with a large number of requests, and it can be difficult to prioritize them, since patient reports are usually not related to his medical records.

These significant drawbacks are deprived of the Medical Messenger (MM) system offered by the authors, which, with external similarity to conventional messengers, allows putting in a reasonable scope the process of remote communication between the doctor and the patient:

- MM requires centralized administration, including the correct identification of the patient.

- MM usage agreement includes the rules of communication sessions. For example, a doctor agrees to respond to a patient's question within 24 h while guaranteeing a quick response in an emergency situation. In this case, urgency can be determined both by the patient himself and by objective indications of remote monitoring. Moreover, the warnings of the remote monitoring systems can serve as the basis for the beginning of the session by the doctor.
- MM is tied to both personal remote monitoring systems and PHR.
- MM has an interface for both mobile devices and conventional computers. This allows the doctor to view the patient's documents in a convenient format on a large screen.
- Finally, MM assumes the use of a paid basis for a limited period. Experience shows that even a small subscription fee disciplines users. In addition, after the expiration of the contract, communication between the doctor and the patient is terminated before the conclusion of a new contract.

All this can make MM a convenient and effective tool for interaction between the doctor and the patient in a variety of situations. The future development of interaction of MM to PHR systems seems to be perspective. We expect this exchange of messages will serve as a base of innovative interactive case history, managed not only by physician, but by patient as well.

The connecting MM to PHR and respond to alarms from remote monitoring devices, supplying the physician with effective tools for analyzing patient data. But there is also a much broader view of this problem: the use of various intelligent algorithms for analyzing medical data. Such algorithms have evolved a long time ago, and were born before computers. Well-known "temperature sheet" allows you to consolidate many data on the patient's condition and to give the doctor the material for a deeper analysis [11, 12]. The

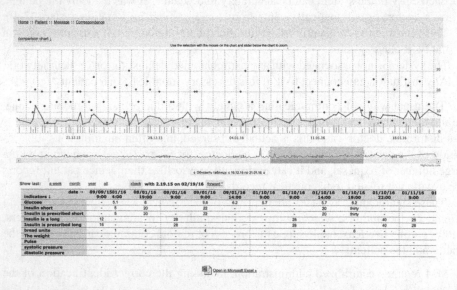

Fig. 1. Distant Monitoring of Pregnant with diabetes. Scalable representation of self-monitoring blood sugar level, amount of carbohydrates in food and insulin doses on WWW.MEDARHIV.RU.

author's team has many years of experience using such algorithms in real clinical conditions [13, 14]. Today graphical integration of medical data can be represented as Scalable Single Time Axe Multimedia Internet-Based Instrument (Fig. 1).

Timely adoption of clinical decisions in pregnant women is possible when using the service of a personal electronic medical service "WWW.MEDARHIV.RU" with a mobile application.

The service provides storage of self-monitoring results, provision to their authorized physician in the form of an integrated schedule of all monitored parameters on a common time axis and calculation of insulin boluses. The patient enters the blood glucose level in the mobile application, the number of "Bread units" (amount of carbohydrates) in the planned meal. Based on the target values, the carbohydrate ratio and the sensitivity factor, which the doctor determines, the program calculates a short-acting insulin dose. In addition, the program provides a reminder function for measuring blood glucose levels, the introduction of insulin and other parameters. An authorized physician can view the information in accordance with the monitoring plan, and off-schedule - at the request of a pregnant woman or an alarm that is generated automatically, according to the settings that the doctor makes.

Test monitoring was performed in 20 pregnant patients with diabetes mellitus. Doctors noted the convenience and effectiveness of remote monitoring: viewing a diary of self-monitoring, nutrition and adjusting insulin therapy on line.

An important advantage of the method was the work with the diabetes for the first time established during pregnancy: the use of the service allowed in a short time to teach pregnant women self-monitoring and evaluate the effectiveness of diet therapy, to carry out, correct and decide on the appointment of insulin.

3 Conclusion

Engaging patients in managing their health, empowering physicians with tools for interacting with patients and analyzing their condition is the central challenges for the entire medical informatics area. It's 10 years (since 2007), then we started PHR service WWW.MEDARHIV.RU and only now its acceptance start to raise quickly (from 5.000 to 100.000 registered users in RF in one year, announced as National service in Kazakhstan).

Acknowledgements. This work was supported, in part, by a Grants RFBR, Russia № 16-29-12998, 16-07-01140, 16-07-01047.

References

1. Shklovskiy-Kordi, N.E., Zingerman, B., Varticovski, L.: Electronic Health Records (EHR) adapted for clinical trials. J. Clin. Oncol. **29**(15_suppl), 345–346 (2011). e16582
2. Shklovskiy-Kordi, N.E., Zingerman, B.: The protection of personal information and the patient's interests and safety - Russian experience. In: Proceedings ESH, Jerusalem, p. 84 (2010)

3. Gusev, A.V.: Criteria for choosing a medical information system (Rus.). Health Manag. **5**, 38–45 (2010)
4. Shklovskiy-Kordi, N.E., Zingerman, B.: Electronic medical map and the principles of its organization (Rus.). Doct. Inf. Technol. **2**, 37–58 (2013)
5. Zingerman, B.: A personal electronic medical card is a service that is available now (Rus.). Doct. Inf. Technol. **3**, 15–25 (2010)
6. Shklovskiy-Kordi, N.E., Zingerman, B., et al.: Computerized case history - an effective tool for the management of patients and clinical trials. In: Proceedings MIE 2005 ENMI European Notes in Medical Informatics, vol. 1(1), pp. 53–58 (2005)
7. Shklovskiy-Kordi, N.E., Zingerman, B., Vorobiev, A.I.: On telemedicine "patient-doctor". Doct. Inf. Technol. **1**, 61–79 (2017)
8. Shklovskiy-Kordi, N.E., Zingerman, B., Varticovski, L.: Electronic Health Records (EHR) adapted for clinical trials. J. Clin. Oncol. **29**, 256–257 (2011). abstract e16582
9. Goldberg, S., Shklovskiy-Kordi, N.E., Zingerman, B.: Time-oriented multi-image case history - the way to the "disease image analysis". In: VISAPP, Barcelona, Spain, pp. 378–383 (2007)
10. Shklovskiy-Kordi, N.E., Zingerman, B., Karp, V.P., Vorobiov, A.I.: Integrated electronic medical record: tasks and problems. Doct. Inf. Technol. **1**, 24–34 (2015)
11. Shklovskiy-Kordi, N.E., Zingerman, B., et al.: Use of computerized time-sensitive multimedia case presentation for clinical outcome analysis. Blood **98**(1), 768 (2001). abstracts 5450
12. Shklovskiy-Kordi, N.E., Zingerman, B., Goldberg, S., Kremenetzkaia, A., Krol, M., Rivkind, N., Vorobiev, A.: Disease image: a time axis presentation of clinical information. Int. J. Hematol. **67**(1), 290–291 (2000)
13. Shklovskiy-Kordi, N., Zingerman, B., Kobeliacky, V., Gudilina, J., Freidin, J., Goldberg, S., Davis, S.: A time axis Presentation of the clinical and diagnostic information from multiple sources. J. Am. Assoc. Med. Inf. Supplement, 1161 (1999)
14. Shklovskiy-Kordi, N., Freidin, J., Goldberg, S., Krol, M., Rivkind, N., Zingerman, B., Davis, S.: Standardization for telemedical consultation on a basis of multimedia case history. In: Proceedings, Fourteenth IEEE Symposium on Computer-Based Medical Systems, pp. 535–540 (2001)

Developing a Tunable Q-Factor Wavelet Transform Based Algorithm for Epileptic EEG Feature Extraction

Hadi Ratham Al Ghayab[1]([✉]), Yan Li[1], Siuly[2], Shahab Abdulla[3], and Paul Wen[1]

[1] Faculty of Health, Engineering and Sciences, University of Southern Queensland,
Darling Heights, QLD 4350, Australia
{HadiRathamGhayab.AlGhayab,Yan.Li,paul.wen}@usq.edu.au
[2] Centre for Applied Informatics, College of Engineering and Science,
Victoria University, Melbourne, Australia
siuly.siuly@vu.edu.au
[3] Open Access College, Language Centre, University of Southern Queensland,
Darling Heights, QLD 4350, Australia
Shahab.Abdulla@usq.edu.au

Abstract. Brain signals refer to electroencephalogram (EEG) data that contain the most important information in the human brain, which are non-stationary and nonlinear in nature. EEG signals are a mixture of sustained oscillation and non-oscillatory transients that are difficult to deal with by linear methods. This paper proposes a new technique based on a tunable Q-factor wavelet transform (TQWT) and statistical method (SM), denoted as TQWT-SM, to analyze epileptic EEG recordings. Firstly, EEG signals are decomposed into different sub—bands by the TWQT method, which is parameterized by its Q-factor and redundancy. This approach depends on the resonance of signals, instead of frequency or scales as the Fourier and wavelet transforms do. Secondly, each type of the sub-band vector is divided into n windows, and 10 statistical features from each window are extracted. Finally all the obtained statistical features are forwarded to a k nearest neighbor (k-NN) classifier to evaluate the performance of the proposed TQWT-SM method. The TQWT-SM features extraction method achieves good experimental results for the seven different epileptic EEG binary-categories by the k-NN classifier, in terms of accuracy (Acc), Matthew's correlation coefficient (MCC), and F score *(F1)*. The outcomes of the proposed technique can assist the experts to detect epileptic seizures.

Keywords: Electroencephalography (EEG) · Tunable Q-factor wavelet transform · Statistical method · k nearest neighbor

1 Introduction

Electroencephalography (EEG) is a significant test to study human brain electrical activities. EEG signals are obtained from electrodes inserted intra-cranially or on the scalp [1]. Analyzing EEG signals is a very challenging task due to their oscillatory and non-oscillatory transients [2], nonlinear, aperiodic, and non-stationary dynamic behaviors. It is really hard to extract the most representative information from a huge size of

© Springer International Publishing AG 2017
S. Siuly et al. (Eds.): HIS 2017, LNCS 10594, pp. 45–55, 2017.
https://doi.org/10.1007/978-3-319-69182-4_6

EEG data for classification. Generally two types of feature extraction methods, linear and nonlinear, are used [3] for EEG classification.

The Fourier and wavelet transforms have been widely used for time series analysis to detect epileptiforms in EEG signals. The Fourier transform is used to transform EEG signals from time series into frequency domain. The most discriminative features in that domain are extracted [4–6]. The Wavelet transform is often applied to EEG data in order to extract the best features from different bands of wavelets [7–11]. In addition to the Fourier and wavelet transforms, other techniques are also utilized for detecting epileptic seizures because EEGs are a mixture of sustained oscillation and non-oscillatory transients that make the EEGs nonlinear and chaotic signals [1–3, 11].

Other nonlinear methods have been applied to extract features in the EEG recordings. A Lyapunov exponent was implemented to extract most significant features in EEG data [12–14]. An empirical mode decomposition was also used to explore the representative samples [15]. In addition, many researchers used entropies from EEG signals as the features [9, 16–18]. However, most of the nonlinear approaches are slow for implementation, which makes them difficult to use in real time [2].

Recently, a tunable Q-factor wavelet transform (TQWT) is getting its popularity in brain signal processing [19–21] as it is a flexible and fully discrete wavelet transform that is particularly suitable for analyzing oscillatory signals [22]. Most wavelet transforms are incapable of tuning their Q-factors. The TQWT is able to adjust its Q-factor and has emerged as a powerful tool for oscillatory signals analysis.

This paper presents a fast and robust nonlinear algorithm to analyze and classify EEG signals. The algorithm is developed based on the tunable Q-factor wavelet transform (TQWT) and a statistical method (SM), denoted as TQWT-SM. K-nearest neighbor (k-NN) is employed to evaluate the performance of the proposed TQWT-SM scheme. The details of this approach are explained in Sects. 2–4. The concluding remarks are provided in Sect. 5.

2 Datasets and Methods

2.1 Experimental Data

This study uses a benchmark EEG database which was collected by Bonn University, Germany, and this database is publicly available[1]. The database contains five different EEG sets. Sets **A** and **B** are recorded from five healthy people with eyes opened and closed, respectively. Sets **C-E** were from different five patients with each set from one subject. Sets **C** and **D** were obtained from epileptic patients with seizures free.

The last set (set **E**) was taken from epileptic subjects during active seizures. Each dataset contained 100 channels with each channel having 4096 observations. Each set contains 23.6 s of data points [23, 24].

---

[1] http://www.meb.unibonn.de/epileptologie/science/physik/eegdata.html.

2.2   Methodology

This section presents a detailed description of the proposed scheme. Figure 1 shows the structure of the proposed TQWT-SM method. The TQWT-SM is used to extract more discriminative features for EEG classification. In order to evaluate the proposed method, k-NN is applied for classification.

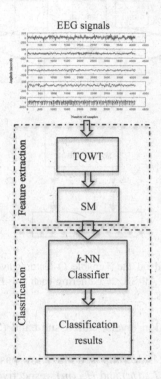

Fig. 1. Block diagram of the proposed scheme for the analysis and classification of EEGs.

Feature extraction: The EEG recordings often include a huge number of data points. Some of those data are redundant, which leads to slowing down the classification process and sometime causes inaccurate results. Feature extraction techniques are often used to reduce the data dimensionality and for a better performance. Figure 2 shows the feature extraction process used in this paper. The following sections explain more details about the method in this study.

Tunable Q-factor wavelet transform (TQWT): The TQWT approach is used to analyze EEG signals based on Q-factor (Q), redundancy (R), and the level of decompositions (J) parameters. The parameters are changeable. The TQWT is an analogous form of the rational-dilation wavelet transform [25, 26], and it has been used to analyze EEG signals [19, 27].

For the TQWT parameters, Q is often set at a high value because EEG signals have more oscillations with low frequency. The TQWT decomposed each EEG channel signal

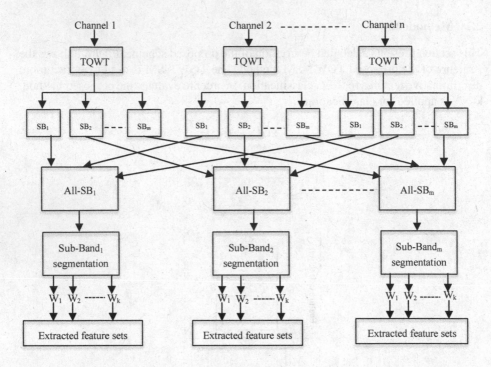

Fig. 2. Feature extraction based on the Tunable Q-factor wavelet transform and statistical method. Note: SB = Sub-Bands; All-SB$_m$ = gathering each Sub-Band from all channels in one set; W$_k$ = the number of windows.

into a number of decomposition levels, called sub-band (SB), using the same input parameters (Q, R, and J).

For each channel signal, it is decomposed into a low pass sub-band and a high pass sub-band, that are denoted as $L_{sig}(m)$ and $H_{sig}(m)$, respectively, at one level of decomposition. The high pass sub-band $H_{sig}(m-1)$ is further decomposed into its low pass sub-band and its high pass sub-band. In this research, the level of decomposition is set at 5. The five levels of sub-bands are calculated using Eqs. (1) and (2) [20, 21, 26]:

$$L_{sig}(m) = \begin{cases} 1, & \text{if } |\omega| \le H_{sig}(m-1)\pi, \\ \theta\left(\dfrac{\omega + H_{sig}(m-1)\pi}{L_{sig}(m) + H_{sig}(m-1)}\right), & \text{if } H_{sig}(m-1)\pi < |\omega| < L_{sig}(m)\pi, \\ 0, & \text{if } L_{sig}(m)\pi \le |\omega| \le \pi, \end{cases} \qquad (1)$$

where $1 =< m <= 5$ is the level of the current decomposition. $H_{sig}(m)$ can be mathematically expressed as [21, 25]:

$$H_{sig}(m) = \begin{cases} 0, & \text{if} \quad |\omega| \leq H_{sig}(m-1)\pi, \\ \theta\left(\dfrac{L_{sig}(m)\pi - \omega}{L_{sig}(m) + H_{sig}(m-1)}\right), & \text{if} \quad H_{sig}(m-1)\pi < |\omega| < L_{sig}(m)\pi, \\ 1, & \text{if} \quad L_{sig}(m)\pi \leq |\omega| \leq \pi, \end{cases} \quad (2)$$

where $\theta(\omega)$ refers to Daubechies filter frequency response and ω is a signal [21, 26]. The values of R, Q, and J in the TQWT are linked to the filter bank parameters, $L_{sig}(m)$ and $H_{sig}(m)$, as in the formulas below [21]:

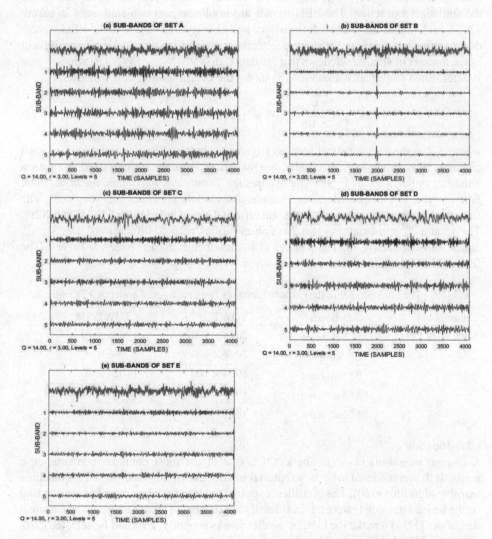

Fig. 3. (a) Plot of set **A** and its Sub-Bands; (b) Plot of set **B** and its Sub-Bands; (c) Plot of set **C** and its Sub-Bands; (d) Plot of set **D** and its Sub-Bands; (e) Plot of set **E** and its Sub-Bands, that are obtained by using TQWT.

$$Q = H_{sig}(m-2)/H_{sig}(m) \tag{3}$$

$$R = H_{sig}(m)/L_{sig}(m-1) \tag{4}$$

The value of Q in this study was set as 14, and R was chosen as 3, while the decompose level J was selected empirically as 5 (for five sub-bands). Figures 3(a)-(e) present a single channel EEG signals from sets **A-E**, and their five sub-bands obtained by the TQWT.

Statistical method (SM): The SM method includes two stages, the segmentation and the statistical extraction. The EEG signals are nonlinear and non-stationary in nature [28], which makes them difficult to analyze and classify. In order to make EEG signals quasi-stationary, firstly, a segmentation technique is utilized to divide each sub-band into a number of smaller windows that are denoted as W_1, W_2,...., W_n. The window size is determined empirically. Equation (5) shows the determination of n windows.

$$S_{feat} = \frac{SB_{chan}}{W}; \quad W = 1, 2, \ldots \ldots, n \tag{5}$$

where S_{feat} = the key statistical features from one window, SB_{chan} = Sub-bands of each channel, W = n-windows. Secondly, ten statistical features are extracted from each window, and denoted as F_SB. The features are {*minimum, maximum, mean, median, first quartile, second quartile, range, standard deviation, skewness, and variance*}. The statistical features can represent important information included in the EEG signals [29]. The 1st and 2nd sub-bands contain 2048 observations with 40 dimensions. The 3rd, 4th, and 5th sub-bands have 1024 data points of 40 dimensions as can be seen in Table 1. The features are forwarded to the k-NN classifier.

Table 1. The total number of the extracted features from each set of epileptic EEG signals.

Datasets	Sub-Bands	TQWT	TQWT-SM
Each set of EEG (A-E)	1st Sub-band	2048×100	2048×40
	2nd Sub-band	2048×100	2048×40
	3rd Sub-band	1024×100	1024×40
	4th Sub-band	1024×100	1024×40
	5th Sub-band	1024×100	1024×40

Classification

K nearest neighbors (k-NN): The k-NN is one of the most common nonparametric methods. It is considered to be the simplest (but effective) method among all the machine learning algorithms [30]. The classifier is applied to classify the extracted features based on the nearest training features. It can classify the unlabeled input features to its k nearest neighbors [31]. To make the k-NN classifier works properly, k should be selected carefully [30–32]. In this paper, $k = 1$ is used.

3   Performance Measurements

In this paper, several measurements were used for evaluating the performance of the proposed TQWT-SM scheme. The n-fold cross validation method was used. The data-sets were divided into n subsets/folds [33, 34]. In each implementation, one fold is used as a testing set and $n - 1$ folds are utilized as a training set. An average accuracy is obtained for the whole process in the cross validation method. 5-fold cross validation is used in this study.

The performance of the proposed method is evaluated using the accuracy rate. The accuracy is defined as the percentage of the correctly classified ones by the classifier for the testing dataset as shown in Eq. (6) [24]:

$$Accuracy = \frac{\sum True\ positives + \sum True\ negatives}{\sum All\ samples} \times 100 \qquad (6)$$

Another statistical measurement method used in this study was F score (F1). This measurement takes into consideration of both the precision and the recall of the test to figure out the score, and the best score is 1 [35]:

$$F1 = \frac{2 \sum True\ positives}{2 \sum True\ positives + \sum False\ positives + \sum False\ negative} \times 100 \qquad (7)$$

Matthew's correlation coefficient (MCC) was also applied in this study to evaluate the performance of the algorithm. The MCC considers true positives (TP), true negatives (TN), false positives (FP), and false negatives (FN) of the test to obtain a result and a significant prediction is 1 [20, 36]. The MCC is defined as below:

$$MCC = \frac{(TP \times TN) - (FP \times FN)}{\sqrt{(TP + FP)(TP + FN)(TN + FP)(TN + FN)}} \times 100 \qquad (8)$$

4   Experimental Results and Discussions

All the five sets of epileptic EEG datasets described in Subsect. 2.1 were used in the paper. The proposed new technique was applied to analyze and extract the key features from the epileptic EEG signals. The TQWT based on the SM was implemented. In order to decompose the epileptic EEG signals into five sub-bands and extract the most repre-sentative features, firstly, the TQWT nonlinear method was applied to each channel of EEG signals.

This method processed the EEG signals based on the resonance of five sub-bands. Secondly, each sub-band from each channel was merged together as a sub-band vector. The sub-band vector was then segmented into a number of windows and ten statistical features were extracted from each window.

The key statistical features were forwarded to the k-NN to evaluate the performance of the proposed approach. Seven different EEG pairs were tested in the experiments.

Table 2 shows the experimental results. In Table 2, all the experimental cases were binary classification except the cases of No. 6 and No. 7, which were multi-classification.

Table 2. The number of EEG pairs in the paper.

No	Case	Descriptions
1	A vs E	Healthy eyes open vs seizures
2	B vs E	Healthy eyes close vs seizures
3	C vs E	Seizures free vs seizures
4	D vs E	Seizures free vs seizures
5	A vs C	Healthy vs seizures free
6	AB vs E	{Healthy eyes open and close} vs seizures
7	A vs CDE	Healthy vs Epileptic patients

Table 3 presents the overall classification accuracies that were yielded by the k-NN. In Table 3, the TQWT-SM method based on the k-NN classifier achieved a 98.5% and 99.3% average classification rate in the five-fold cross validation for the pairs of {A vs E} and {AB vs E}, respectively, in the 5th sub-band. A 98.9%, 98.4%, and 98.6% average accuracy for the cases of NO. 2, 3, 4, respectively, obtained in the 1st sub-band by the TQWT-SM.

Table 3. The accuracies (Acc) for the five sub-bands by the TQWT-SM method

No	Case	Classifier	Average accuracy (%)				
			1st	2nd	3rd	4th	5th
1	A vs E	k-NN	98.2	96.8	97.6	96.1	98.5
2	B vs E	k-NN	98.9	98.4	97.3	96.2	98.7
3	C vs E	k-NN	98.4	95.9	97.2	94.9	97.2
4	D vs E	k-NN	98.6	97.3	96.1	96.6	98.3
5	A vs C	k-NN	87.2	90.4	88.2	84.7	86.7
6	AB vs E	k-NN	98.6	97.5	98.5	97.8	99.3
7	A vs CDE	k-NN	87.9	91.0	88.5	84.6	87.4

On the other hand, the technique yielded a 90.4% and 91% overall classification accuracy for the cases of (healthy vs seizure free) and (healthy vs epileptic patients), respectively. Those two groups were more similar to each other, which caused the lowest classification accuracy compared to other cases. Clearly, in terms of the accuracy, the TQWT-SM with the k-NN classifier achieved good results.

Tables 4 and 5 show the average results for the MCC and $F1$ in the five-fold cross validation. Those results were achieved by the TQWT-SM and the k-NN classifier. As presented in Tables 3, 4 and 5, the TQWT-SM can provide good accuracy, MCC and $F1$ score through the k-NN classifier in the 1st, 2nd, and 5th sub-bands.

Table 4. The average MCC for the five sub-bands by the TQWT-SM method

No	Case	Classifier	MCC (%)				
			1st	2nd	3rd	4th	5th
1	A vs E	k-NN	96.29	93.90	94.50	93.07	97.08
2	B vs E	k-NN	97.80	96.89	94.11	91.81	96.78
3	C vs E	k-NN	96.68	92.16	94.68	89.55	95.31
4	D vs E	k-NN	97.12	94.78	91.72	94.15	96.68
5	A vs C	k-NN	73.88	81.35	77.74	67.82	74.01
6	AB vs E	k-NN	96.30	94.71	96.79	94.78	98.24
7	A vs CDE	k-NN	67.48	75.90	69.40	58.52	66.46

Table 5. The average *F1* score for the five sub-bands by TQWT-SM method

No	Case	Classifier	F1 (%)				
			1st	2nd	3rd	4th	5th
1	A vs E	k-NN	98.20	97.14	97.31	96.27	98.78
2	B vs E	k-NN	98.88	98.33	97.17	96.01	98.59
3	C vs E	k-NN	98.08	96.35	97.59	94.50	97.76
4	D vs E	k-NN	98.56	97.40	95.89	97.08	98.34
5	A vs C	k-NN	87.16	90.72	89.10	84.18	87.27
6	AB vs E	k-NN	98.77	98.26	98.94	98.28	99.42
7	A vs CDE	k-NN	75.52	81.92	77.05	68.88	74.96

5   Conclusions

This paper proposed a new methodology for epileptic EEG feature extraction. The key features were extracted from the five sub-bands after applying the TQWT-SM, and were forwarded to the popular k-NN classifier. The performance of the proposed technique was evaluated through the accuracy, Mathew's correlation coefficient and the F score. The experimental results showed that the TQWT-SM with the k-NN classifier was able to discriminate the epileptic EEG signals with a satisfactory performance. The TQWT-SM method can help the experts to analyze a large volume of EEG data. In the future, the proposed technique will be adapted to analyze and classify other EEG signals.

References

1. Siuly, S., Li, Y., Wen, P.: Analysis and classification of EEG signals using a hybrid clustering technique. In: 2010 IEEE/ICME International Conference on Complex Medical Engineering (CME), pp. 34–39. IEEE (2010)
2. Selesnick, I.W.: Resonance-based signal decomposition: a new sparsity-enabled signal analysis method. Sig. Process. **91**(12), 2793–2809 (2011)
3. Zhu, G., Li, Y., Wen, P.P.: Epileptic seizure detection in EEGs signals using a fast weighted horizontal visibility algorithm. Comput. Methods Programs Biomed. **115**(2), 64–75 (2014)

4. Kohtoh, S., Taguchi, Y., Matsumoto, N., Wada, M., Huang, Z.L., Urade, Y.: Algorithm for sleep scoring in experimental animals based on fast Fourier transform power spectrum analysis of the electroencephalogram. Sleep Biol. Rhythms **6**(3), 163–171 (2008)

5. Polat, K., Güneş, S.: Classification of epileptiform EEG using a hybrid system based on decision tree classifier and fast Fourier transform. Appl. Math. Comput. **187**(2), 1017–1026 (2007)

6. Murugappan, M., Murugappan, S., Gerard, C.: Wireless EEG signals based neuromarketing system using Fast Fourier Transform (FFT). In: 2014 IEEE 10th International Colloquium on Signal Processing & its Applications (CSPA), pp. 25–30. IEEE (2014)

7. Samar, V.J., Bopardikar, A., Rao, R., Swartz, K.: Wavelet analysis of neuroelectric waveforms: a conceptual tutorial. Brain Lang. **66**(1), 7–60 (1999)

8. Subasi, A., Alkan, A., Koklukaya, E., Kiymik, M.K.: Wavelet neural network classification of EEG signals by using AR model with MLE preprocessing. Neural Networks **18**(7), 985–997 (2005)

9. Zhang, Y., Liu, B., Ji, X., Huang, D.: Classification of EEG signals based on autoregressive model and wavelet packet decomposition. Neural Process. Lett. **45**(2), 1–14 (2016)

10. Lekshmi, S., Selvam, V., Rajasekaran, M.P.: EEG signal classification using Principal Component Analysis and Wavelet Transform with Neural Network. In: 2014 International Conference on Communications and Signal Processing (ICCSP), pp. 687–690. IEEE (2014)

11. Gajic, D., Djurovic, Z., Di Gennaro, S., Gustafsson, F.: Classification of EEG signals for detection of epileptic seizures based on wavelets and statistical pattern recognition. Biomed. Eng. Appl. Basis Commun. **26**(02), 1450021 (2014)

12. Pritchard, W.S., Duke, D.W., Krieble, K.K.: Dimensional analysis of resting human EEG II: surrogate-data testing indicates nonlinearity but not low-dimensional chaos. Psychophysiology **32**(5), 486–491 (1995)

13. Adeli, H., Ghosh-Dastidar, S., Dadmehr, N.: A wavelet-chaos methodology for analysis of EEGs and EEG subbands to detect seizure and epilepsy. IEEE Trans. Biomed. Eng. **54**(2), 205–211 (2007)

14. Hosseinifard, B., Moradi, M.H., Rostami, R.: Classifying depression patients and normal subjects using machine learning techniques and nonlinear features from EEG signal. Comput. Methods Programs Biomed. **109**(3), 339–345 (2013)

15. Acharya, U.R., Sudarshan, V.K., Adeli, H., Santhosh, J., Koh, J.E., Puthankatti, S.D., Adeli, A.: A novel depression diagnosis index using nonlinear features in EEG signals. Eur. Neurol. **74**(1–2), 79–83 (2015)

16. Pachori, R.B., Patidar, S.: Epileptic seizure classification in EEG signals using second-order difference plot of intrinsic mode functions. Comput. Methods Programs Biomed. **113**(2), 494–502 (2014)

17. Broberg, R., Lewis, R.: Classification of epileptoid oscillations in EEG using Shannon's entropy amplitude probability distribution. In: Traina, A.J.M., Traina, C., Cordeiro, R.L.F. (eds.) SISAP 2014. LNCS, vol. 8821, pp. 247–252. Springer, Cham (2014). doi: 10.1007/978-3-319-11988-5_23

18. Jie, X., Cao, R., Li, L.: Emotion recognition based on the sample entropy of EEG. Bio-Med. Mater. Eng. **24**(1), 1185–1192 (2014)

19. Patidar, S., Pachori, R.B., Upadhyay, A., Acharya, U.R.: An integrated alcoholic index using tunable-Q wavelet transform based features extracted from EEG signals for diagnosis of alcoholism. Appl. Soft Comput. **50**, 71–78 (2017)

20. Patidar, S., Panigrahi, T.: Detection of epileptic seizure using Kraskov entropy applied on tunable-Q wavelet transform of EEG signals. Biomed. Signal Process. Control **34**, 74–80 (2017)

21. Patidar, S., Pachori, R.B., Acharya, U.R.: Automated diagnosis of coronary artery disease using tunable-Q wavelet transform applied on heart rate signals. Knowl.-Based Syst. **82**, 1–10 (2015)
22. Hassan, A.R., Siuly, S., Zhang, Y.: Epileptic seizure detection in EEG signals using tunable-Q factor wavelet transform and bootstrap aggregating. Comput. Methods Programs Biomed. **137**, 247–259 (2016)
23. Andrzejak, R.G., Lehnertz, K., Mormann, F., Rieke, C., David, P., Elger, C.E.: Indications of nonlinear deterministic and finite-dimensional structures in time series of brain electrical activity: Dependence on recording region and brain state. Phys. Rev. E **64**(6), 061907 (2001)
24. Al Ghayab, H.R., Li, Y., Abdulla, S., Diykh, M., Wan, X.: Classification of epileptic EEG signals based on simple random sampling and sequential feature selection. Brain Inform. **3**(2), 85–91 (2016)
25. Bayram, I., Selesnick, I.W.: Frequency-domain design of overcomplete rational-dilation wavelet transforms. IEEE Trans. Signal Process. **57**(8), 2957–2972 (2009)
26. Selesnick, I.W.: Wavelet transform with tunable Q-factor. IEEE Trans. Signal Process. **59**(8), 3560–3575 (2011)
27. Bhattacharyya, A., Pachori, R.B., Upadhyay, A., Acharya, U.R.: Tunable-Q wavelet transform based multiscale entropy measure for automated classification of Epileptic EEG signals. Appl. Sci. **7**(4), 385 (2017)
28. Nguyen-Ky, T., Wen, P., Li, Y., Malan, M.: Measuring the hypnotic depth of anaesthesia based on the EEG signal using combined wavelet transform, eigenvector and normalisation techniques. Comput. Biol. Med. **42**(6), 680–691 (2012)
29. Siuly, S., Kabir, E., Wang, H., Zhang, Y.: Exploring sampling in the detection of multicategory EEG signals. In: Computational and Mathematical Methods in Medicine 2015 (2015)
30. Duda, R.O., Hart, P.E., Stork, D.G.: Pattern Classification. Wiley, New York (2012)
31. Ergen, B.: Scale invariant and fixed-length feature extraction by integrating discrete cosine transform and autoregressive signal modeling for palmprint identification. Turk. J. Electr. Eng. Comput. Sci. **24**(3), 1768–1781 (2016)
32. Cover, T., Hart, P.: Nearest neighbor pattern classification. IEEE Trans. Inf. Theory **13**(1), 21–27 (1967)
33. Siuly, S., Li, Y.: Designing a robust feature extraction method based on optimum allocation and principal component analysis for epileptic EEG signal classification. Comput. Methods Programs Biomed. **119**(1), 29–42 (2015)
34. Siuly, S., Li, Y., Wen, P.: Identification of motor imagery tasks through CC–LR algorithm in brain computer interface. Int. J. Bioinform. Res. Appl. **9**(2), 156–172 (2013)
35. Powers, D.M.: Evaluation: from precision, recall and F-measure to ROC, informedness, markedness and correlation. J. Mach. Learn. Technol. **2**(1), 37–63 (2011)
36. Azar, A.T., El-Said, S.A.: Performance analysis of support vector machines classifiers in breast cancer mammography recognition. Neural Comput. Appl. **24**(5), 1163–1177 (2014)

Granular Computing Combined with Support Vector Machines for Diagnosing Erythemato-Squamous Diseases

Yongchao Wang[1,2] and Juanying Xie[3(✉)]

[1] Information Science and Technology, Aichi Prefrctural University,
Nagakute, Aichi 480-1198, Japan
[2] School of Computer Science and Engineering, Xi'an University of Technology,
Xi'an 710048, People's Republic of China
[3] School of Computer Science, Shaanxi Normal University,
Xi'an 710062, People's Republic of China
xiejuany@snnu.edu.cn

Abstract. A computational model with a new hybrid feature selection approach is developed in this paper to determine the type of erythemato-squamous disease. The new feature selection method combines the strength of granular computing (GrC) and support vector machines (SVM) together with the advantages of filters and wrappers to select the optimal feature subset to build a sound classifier. We treat the erythemato-squamous disease dataset as a decision information system, where the sample features are considered as condition attributes and the class label the decision attribute. We calculate the granular of each feature and decision attribute, then evaluate the significance of each feature to classification by the difference between its granularity and that of decision attribute, after that we rank features in descending order by their significance. Generalized sequential forward search (GSFS) strategy together with SVM is adopted to select the necessary features to condense decision information system without compromising its classification capacity. 5-fold cross validation experiments have been conducted on the erythemato-squamous disease dataset taken from UCI (University of California Irvine) machine learning repository. Experimental results demonstrate that our diagnostic model has got condensed decision information system for erythemato-squamous disease with less features than the original ones while achieving a comparable accuracy in the literature.

Keywords: Granular computing · Support vector machines · Feature selection · Erythemato-squamous diseases · Rough sets · Decision information systems

1 Introduction

Erythemato-squamous diseases are frequently seen in outpatient dermatology departments [7,8]. The diagnosis for the diseases is very challenging because the six groups of them including psoriasis, seboreic dermatitis, lichen planus,

© Springer International Publishing AG 2017
S. Siuly et al. (Eds.): HIS 2017, LNCS 10594, pp. 56–68, 2017.
https://doi.org/10.1007/978-3-319-69182-4_7

pityriasis rosea, chronic dermatitis and pityriasis rubra pilaris share the clinical features of erythema with very few differences. A biopsy is usually necessary to diagnose these diseases, but they almost share the same histopathological features. The other difficulty for the differential diagnosis is that one disease may show the histopathological characteristics of another ones at the initial stage and may have got its own ones at the following stages, and some samples may show the typical histopathological features of the disease while some others do not. Patients are often first diagnosed according to the 12 clinical features. Then the skin samples are taken for the evaluation of 22 histopathological features. The values of these 22 histopathological features are determined by the analysis of samples under a microscope [7]. The most difficult for diagnosing the diseases is that the pathogenesises of the diseases are not known.

Many experts in artificial intelligence field devote themselves to studying the automatic diagnoses methods of erythemato-squamous diseases, and there has been much work in the area. These works can be classified three categories. One is the ones that focus on finding the efficient machine learning methods to diagnose erythemato-squamous by its features [18, 19, 23, 25–28, 30]. The second is the ones that introduce the feature selection methods to delete the irrelevant or redundant features to detect the very distinguishable features to comprise the feature subset to construct the diagnostic model to make an efficient and sound diagnosing for erythemato-squamous diseases [1, 12, 16, 24, 34–37]. The last is another trend which introduces the unsupervised learning techniques to classify the erythemato-squamous diseases effectively [29, 39].

It is always the fact that there are several features redundant or irrelative to diagnosis erythemato-squamous diseases. It has been proved that all of the features are not important for a specific task [2, 11]. Feature selection plays and important role to delete this kind of features and preserve the essential ones, so that it has become an important preprocessing step in constructing an efficient and effective model to diagnosis erythemato-squamous diseases [1, 12, 16, 24, 34–37].

Granular Computing (GrC) is a new trend in artificial intelligence field and it is derived from rough sets theory (RST). GrC has the capability to describe a real world problem in different level granularities, thereby it can abstract a problem at different level of abstraction [14]. GrC has been proved to be the powerful tool to solve the problem with some uncertain properties. It has become one of the very popular mathematic tools in artificial intelligence. GrC can combine the clustering and feature selection problems together to some extent, and it has been demonstrated to possess many distinguishable properties. In addition, support vector machine (SVM) is one of best classification tools with very good generalization and minimum structure risk [22, 31]. Therefore we combine the strength of GrC and SVM in this study to develop a new feature selection method as the preprocess to construct an efficient model to diagnose erythemato-squamous diseases, where GrC performs feature selection, SVM is a classification tool to guide the feature selection procedure according to the classification accuracy of the specific SVM classifier based on the specific feature subset.

This paper is organized as follows. Section 2 reviews the primary theories used in our study, including the key concepts of GrC and SVM. Section 3 describes our GrC and SVM based hybrid feature selection algorithm. Section 4 demonstrates the experimental results and the analysis. Finally, Sect. 5 draws conclusions and describes future work.

2   The Basic Knowledge of GrC and SVM

2.1   The Basic Idea of GrC

GrC was coined by Lin [14]. It is the generalization of RST and the neighborhood system. GrC represents the real world problems in a specific level of granularity, and it can model the real world problems in multiple levels. GrC is a kind of methodology that partitions the universe of a problem into different granules based on the indiscernibility relation between samples of the universe, as a consequence it can express a problem precisely. GrC has become a powerful tool to deal with uncertain or vague or incomplete information systems. It provides a conceptual framework for studying the issues in data mining, machine learning, clustering analysis and many other areas in artificial intelligence. There are three models in GrC including rough sets model, fuzzy set model and entropy space model [38]. Here are the basic concepts of GrC [20].

Definition 1. Let $K = (U, \Re)$ be a knowledge base, and $R \in \Re$ the equivalence relation on the domain U, then the partition U/R is called a knowledge of U. We often use R to denote the knowledge U/R. The granularity of knowledge R, denoted by $GD(R)$, is: $GD(R) = \frac{\|R\|}{\|U \times U\|} = \frac{\|R\|}{\|U\|^2}$. So if $U/R = \{X_1, X_2, \cdots, X_n\}$, then $GD(R) = \sum_{i=1}^{n} \frac{\|X_i\|^2}{\|U\|^2}$.

Definition 1 tells us that the granularity of knowledge R describes its discrimination. That is, for $\forall u, v \in U$, if $(u, v) \in R$, then u, v are indistinguishable according to R, because they belong to the same equivalence group of R. Otherwise, they can be distinguishable. It is obvious that $GD(R)$ means the degree of the indiscrimination of two objects in U according to the knowledge R of it. The bigger the $GD(R)$ is, the less discriminability the knowledge R is.

Definition 2. Let R be a knowledge of knowledge base $K = (U, \Re)$, and $U/R = \{X_1, X_2, \cdots, X_n\}$, then the distinguishability of R denoted as $Dis(R)$ is: $Dis(R) = 1 - GD(R) = 1 - \sum_{i=1}^{n} \frac{\|X_i\|^2}{\|U\|^2}$

It is obvious that the bigger the $Dis(R)$ is, the stronger the distinguishability is the knowledge R.

Property 1. Let R be a knowledge of knowledge base $K = (U, \Re)$, then the followings hold. $\frac{1}{\|U\|} \leq GD(R) \leq 1, 0 \leq Dis(R) \leq 1 - \frac{1}{\|U\|}$.

Definition 3. Let $S = \langle U, A, V, f \rangle$ be an information system, and $P \subseteq A$ be a subset of attributes, and $p \in A - P$ an attribute. Then we use $Sig_P(p)$ to denote the significance of p to P. That is, $Sig_P(p) = 1 - \frac{\|P \bigcup \{p\}\|}{\|P\|}$, where $\|P\| = card(IND(P))$.

If $U/IND(P) = U/P = \{X_1, X_2, \cdots, X_n\}$, then $\|P\| = \sum\limits_{i=1}^{n} \|X_i\|^2$. $Sig_P(p)$ expresses the increase in the discrimination of knowledge P when the attribute p is added to P.

It is obvious that the bigger the $Sig_P(p)$ is, the more importance is the attribute p to P. If $P = \Phi$, then $Sig_P(p)$ is simplified as $Sig(p)$. That is, $Sig(p) = 1 - \frac{\|p\|}{\|U\|^2}$. So it is obvious that $0 \leq Sig(p) \leq 1 - \frac{1}{\|U\|}$ holds.

Theorem 1. Let $S = \langle U, A, V, f \rangle$ be an information system, $p \in A$ be an attribute. Then the significance of p equals its discriminability. That is, $Sig(p) = Dis(p) = 1 - GD(p)$.

2.2   Support Vector Machines

SVM, developed by Vapnik [31], is a popular machine learning technique. SVM is based on the VC dimension and the structural risk minimization. I has been proved that SVM is superior to the empirical risk minimization. SVM can handle a nonlinear classification problem efficiently by mapping samples from low dimensional input space into high dimensional feature space with a nonlinear kernel function. In feature space, SVM tries to maximize the generalization performance by solving a quadratic programming problem, and then finds the optimal separating hyperplane which is the maximal margin hyperplane. It has been found that SVM is the classification tool with minimum classification error rate and the strongest generalization ability [22]. SVM has been applied to study cancers and many other diseases classifications [9, 23, 27, 34–37] .

Given the training set $\{(x_i, y_i) | x_i \in R^N, \ y_i \in \{-1, 1\}, \ i = 1, \cdots, n\}$, each separating hyperplane qualifies (1) for a binary classification problem.

$$y_i((w \cdot x_i) + b) \geq +1 - \xi_i \tag{1}$$

where $\xi_i \geq 0$ is a slack variable. To find the optimal separating hyperplane, one should minimize (2) subject to (1).

$$\frac{1}{2}\|w\|^2 + C\sum_{i=1}^{n} \xi_i \tag{2}$$

where C is a positive constant parameter to control the tradeoff between the complexity and classification accuracy. By introducing Lagrange multipliers and making appropriate substitutions, minimizing (2) can be substituted by the dual quadratic optimization of (3).

$$
\begin{aligned}
Maxmize \quad & \sum_{i=1}^{n} \dot{\alpha}_i - \tfrac{1}{2} \sum_{i,j=1}^{n} \alpha_i \alpha_j y_i y_j (x_i \cdot x_j) \\
s.t. \quad & \sum_{i=1}^{n} \alpha_i y_i = 0, \ C \geq \alpha_i \geq 0, \ i = 1, \cdots, n
\end{aligned}
\tag{3}
$$

Solving (3), one can get the decision function in (4). For nonlinear case, the decision function in (4) becomes as the equation in (5) using a kernel function to substitute the dot product of data points.

$$
f(x) = sgn(\sum_{i=1}^{n} \alpha_i y_i (x_i \cdot x) + b)
\tag{4}
$$

$$
f(x) = sgn(\sum_{i=1}^{n} \alpha_i y_i K(x_i, x) + b)
\tag{5}
$$

The common kernel functions include: *Linear kernels*: $K(x, x') = x \cdot x'$; *Polynomial kernels*: $K(x, x') = (x \cdot x' + 1)^d$, where d is a positive integer number; *RBF kernels*: $K(x, x') = exp(-\|x - x'\|^2 / \gamma^2)$, where γ is a positive real number.

3   GrC and SVM Based Feature Selection Algorithm

Feature selection plays an important role in building a classification system [5, 6, 9, 10, 15, 17, 32]. It not only reduces the dimensionality of data, but also reduces the computational cost and gains a good classification performance [9]. The general feature selection algorithms comprise two categories: the filters and the wrappers [4, 13]. The filters identify a feature subset from original ones with a given evaluation criterion which is independent of learning algorithms, while the wrappers choose those features with high prediction performance estimated by a specific learning algorithm. The filters are efficient because of its independence to learning algorithms, while wrappers can obtain higher classification accuracy with the deficiency in generalization and computational cost.

This study will combines the advantages of filters and wrappers to present a hybrid feature selection algorithm based on GrC and SVM for diagnosing erythemato-squamous disease. The proposed feature selection algorithm uses GrC as filters to calculate the importance of a feature to classification, and the generalized sequential forward search (GSFS) with SVM as wrappers to evaluate the capability of a feature subset to classfication. We rank features in descending order by their discernibility evaluated by GrC. GSFS strategy is adopted to select the important and necessary features one by one by constructing many temporary SVM classifiers, whilst SVM is used as a classification tool to direct the feature selection procedure.

3.1 Feature search strategies

The basic feature selection strategies include sequential forward search (SFS) proposed by Whitney in [33] and sequential backward search (SBS) presented by Marill *et al.* in [21]. SFS starts by selecting the best single feature, then the best pair is selected where the pair includes the best single feature selected. This process is continued by selecting a single feature that appears to be best when combined with the previously selected feature subset. SBS deletes the worst feature at each iteration where the worst feature is the one without which the remaining ones will get the best performance in classification. To find the worst feature SBS has to try deleting each available feature, which cost the heavy computational cost to SBS. GSFS generalized SFS by selecting the important features one by one according to their ranks, not as SFS selecting the feature that is the best one combined with the selected ones. So GSFS is faster than SFS in feature selection process.

3.2 Search for Best Parameters

To get the optimal diagnostic model for erythemato-squamous diseases, we adopt the grid search technique to discover the best parameter pair (C, γ) for RBF of SVM for each temporary training subset with a specific feature subset, where $log_2 C = \{-5, -4, -3, \cdots, 13, 14, 15\}$, and $log_2 \gamma = \{-15, -13, -11, \cdots, -3, 1, 3\}$. 5-fold cross validation experiments are conducted to train the temporary decision information system for each pair (C, γ). The pair (C, γ) with the highest average training accuracy is considered as the best one and selected to construct the classification model for the temporary decision information system with the specific feature subset.

3.3 GrC Combined SVM Feature Selection Algorithm

In GrC theory, especially the rough sets model, a dataset is called a special information system in which each sample has got its own class label besides its condition features, i.e., a decision information system or a decision table, where the features of a sample, including class label and condition features, are called attributes, such that there are two kinds of attributes, the decision attributes and condition attributes, mapping the class label and the condition features, and there is no overlapping between these two kinds of attributes.

Let $S = \langle U, C \bigcup D, V, f \rangle$ be a decision information system, where C is the set of condition attributes, and D the decision attribute set, then $C \bigcap D = \Phi$. It should be noted that the decision information system we studied here refers to the one which has only one decision attribute.

We combine the strengths of GrC and SVM together to uncover the attribute subset to make the decision information system of erythemato-squamous diseases become as concise as possible without compromising its classification capability. The description of our GrC and SVM based feature selection algorithm is decribed in the following Algorithm 1. It should be noted that kernel function for SVM we used is RBF, and the parameters for the RBF is found by the method described in Subsect. 3.2.

Input: $IS = (U, C, D, V, f)$
Output: the reduction set $RED(C)$
$RED(C) = \Phi$;
calculate $GD(D)$;
for *each* $a \in C$ **do**
$\quad$ calculate $GD(a)$;
$\quad$ calculate $Sig(a)$;
$\quad$ let $Imp(a) = \|sig(a) - sig(D)\|$ *or* $Imp(a) = \|GD(a) - GD(D)\|$;
end
rank condition attributes in descending order according to their Imp values;
let $a = argmaximum\{Imp(a)|a \in C\}$;
let $RED(C) = RED(C) \cup \{a\}$;
CC = C;
while $CC \neq \Phi$ **do**
$\quad$ construct a temporary decision information system with $RED(C)$ and decision attribute;
$\quad$ training a SVM classifier on the training subset via 5-fold cross validation experiment to discover the optimal temporary model;
$\quad$ record the classification accuracy of the optimal model on the training and test subset;
$\quad$ $CC = CC - \{a\}$;
$\quad$ let $a = argmaximum\{Imp(a)|a \in CC\}$;
$\quad$ let $RED(C) = RED(C) \cup \{a\}$;
end
output the best $RED(C)$;
$\quad$ **Algorithm 1.** GrC and SVM combined feature selection algorithm

The best $RED(C)$ is the one that has got the highest training accuracy and with the smallest cardinality as well. The optimal diagnostic model is build on the best reduction. This best reduction $RED(C)$ is the feature subset that we have tried to looking for.

4   Experiments and Results

This section will first describe erythemato-squamous diseases dataset from UCI machine learning repository [3], then display the 5-fold cross validation experimental results and the analysis.

4.1   The Erythemato-Squamous Diseases Dataset

The erythemato-squamous diseases consisting of 366 exemplars with 34 features for each sample and 6 classes in total. There are 8 samples with missing values.

We delete the 8 exemplars in our experiment, so the size of the dataset used is 358. The family history feature in the dataset was given the value 1 if any of the diseases has been observed in the family and 0 otherwise. The age feature simply represents the patient age. Each other feature (clinical and histopathological) was given in a degree of the range from 0 to 3, where, 0 indicates that the feature was not present, 3 indicates the largest amount possible, and 1, 2 indicate the relative intermediate values.

4.2   Experimental Results and Analysis

We try to construct an optimal diagnostic model which can determine the type of erythemato-squamous disease according to its features. We conduct 5-fold cross

Table 1. The average results of 5-fold cross validation experimental results/%

		Feature subset	Sensitivity	Specificity	Accuracy
Fold1	Psoriasis	{ 31, 30, 7, 13,	100.00	98.04	98.65
	Seboreic dermatitis	11, 15, 8, 6,	100.00	100.00	
	Lichen planus	23, 12, 29, 27,	93.33	100.00	
	Pityriasis rosea	25, 33, 24, 26,	100.00	100.00	
	Chronic dermatitis	10, 22, 20, 9,	100.00	100.00	
	Pityriasis rubra pilaris	18, 14, 1, 5 }	100.00	100.00	
Fold1	Psoriasis	{ 31, 30, 7, 13, 11,	100.00	100.00	98.61
	Seboreic dermatitis	15, 8, 6, 12, 23,	91.67	100.00	
	Lichen planus	25, 27, 29, 33, 24,	100.00	100.00	
	Pityriasis rosea	26, 10, 22, 20, 9,	100.00	98.39	
	Chronic dermatitis	14, 18, 1, 5, 17,	100.00	100.00	
	Pityriasis rubra pilaris	2, 32, 28 }	100.00	100.00	
Fold3	Psoriasis	{ 31, 30, 7, 13,	100.00	100.00	98.61
	Seboreic dermatitis	11, 15, 8, 6,	100.00	98.33	
	Lichen planus	23, 12, 27, 29,	100.00	100.00	
	Pityriasis rosea	25, 33, 24, 26,	90.00	100.00	
	Chronic dermatitis	10, 22, 20, 9,	100.00	100.00	
	Pityriasis rubra pilaris	18, 14, 5 }	100.00	100.00	
Fold4	Psoriasis	{ 31, 30, 7, 11,	100.00	100.00	97.14
	Seboreic dermatitis	13, 15, 8, 12,	100.00	96.55	
	Lichen planus	6, 23, 25, 27,	100.00	100.00	
	Pityriasis rosea	29, 24, 33, 26,	77.78	100.00	
	Chronic dermatitis	10, 20, 22, 9,	100.00	100.00	
	Pityriasis rubra pilaris	18, 14, 5 }	100.00	100.00	
Fold5	Psoriasis	{31, 30, 7, 13,	100.00	100.00	100.00
	Seboreic dermatitis	11, 15, 8, 12,	100.00	100.00	
	Lichen planus	6, 25, 27, 29,	100.00	100.00	
	Pityriasis rosea	23, 33, 24, 26,	100.00	100.00	
	Chronic dermatitis	10, 22, 9, 20,	100.00	100.00	
	Pityriasis rubra pilaris	14, 18, 1, 5 }	100.00	100.00	
Average & Intersection size		23	98.43	99.71	98.61

Table 2. Classification accuracies of our algorithm and other available studies

Author	Method	Accuracy/%
Übeyli and Güler (2005)	ANFIS	95.50
Luukka and Leppälampi (2006)	Fuzzy similarity-based classification	97.02
Polat and Günes (2006)	Fuzzy weighted pre-processing	88.18
	K-NN based weighted pre-processing	97.57
	Decision tree	99.00
Nanni (2006)	LSVM	97.22
	RS	97.22
	B1_5	97.50
	B1_10	98.10
	B1_15	97.22
	B2_5	97.50
	B2_10	97.80
	B2_15	98.30
Luukka (2007)	Similarity measure	97.80
Übeyli (2008)	Multiclass SVM with the ECOC	98.32
Polat and Günes (2009)	C4.5 and one-against-all	96.71
Übeylii (2009)	CNN	97.77
Liu et al. (2009)	Naïve Bayes	96.72
	1-NN	92.18
	C4.5	95.08
	PIPPER	92.20
Karabatak and Ince (2009)	AR and NN	98.61
Übeyli and Doğdu (2010)	K-means clustering	94.22
Xie et al. (2011)	IFSFS+SVM	98.61
Xie et al. (2012)	GFSFS+SVM	98.89
	modified GFSFS+SVM	99.17
	GFSFFS+SVM	96.08
	modified GFSFFS+SVM	98.33
	GFSBFS+SVM	95.81
	modified GFSBFS+SVM	95.28
Xie et al. (2013)	two-stage GFSFS	100
	two-stage new GFSFS	100
	two-stage GFSFFS	100
	two-stage new GFSFFS	100
	two-stage GFSBFS	100
	two-stage new GFSBFS	97.06
Özcift and Gülten (2013)	GA+BN	99.20
Abdi and Giveki (2013)	PSO+SVM	98.91
Zhang et al. (2017)	K-means with preprocessing	95.38
This study	Grc+SVM	98.61

validation experiments. The optimal diagnostic model is obtained by training exemplars in training set. The classifier with the lowest training error rate and the smallest size of feature subset is chosen as the optimal diagnostic model.

Then the model is tested by the test subset in terms of classification accuracy, sensitivity and specificity. Table 1 shows the experimental results of the 5-fold cross validation experiments. Table 2 summarizes the classification accuracy of our model and the available studies on diagnosing erythemato-squamous diseases.

It can be seen from the results in Table 1 that the average classification accuracy of the 5-fold cross validation experiments is 98.61%. The model constructed on the feature subset of the 5th fold has got the best performance with the 100% classification accuracy, sensitivity and specificity. The average sensitivity of the 5-fold cross validation experiments is 98.43%, and the average specificity is 99.71%. There are up to 23 features among the maximum 28 selected ones are same in the 5-fold cross validation experiments, but the distinguishability of each feature subset is various, which can be seen from the classification accuracy and the sensitivity and specificity of each fold displayed in Table 1. This fact means that the order of features to be selected will influence the power of the feature subset, and the correlation between features also affects the capability of the feature subset.

The summary in Table 2 demonstrates that our GrC and SVM based hybrid feature selection algorithm can detect the good feature subset on which to build the SVM classification model to diagnose erythemato-squamous diseases. The average classification accuracy of 5-fold cross validation experiment can go up to 98.61%. Although the SVM model we realized cannot whelm the state-of-the-art algorithms for diagnosing erythemato-squamous diseases, it is still a comparable one, and it opened the branch to find the related and important features by GrC for erythemato-squamous diseases.

5   Conclusions

This paper presents a diagnostic model with a new hybrid feature selection algorithm based on GrC and SVM for diagnosing erythemato-squamous diseases. The new hybrid feature selection algorithm combines the strengths of filters and wrappers, where GrC is used as an evaluation criterion of filters, and SVM with GSFS strategy the evaluation system of wrappers to uncover the optimal feature subset with capability to diagnose erythemato-squamous diseases efficiently. 5-fold cross validation experimental results demonstrate the power of our Grc and SVM based feature selection algorithm in selecting the feature subset on which to build the diagnostic model for erythemato-squamous diseases.

However, in order to get a good SVM model, we conducted grid search to get the optimal parameters for each SVM classifier when doing 5-fold cross validation experiment, which incurred extra computation costs. Minimizing the cost for the best optimal parameters of SVM is one of the directions for our future work.

Acknowledgement. We are most grateful to H. Altay Guvenir who created the erythemato-squamous dataset as well as to G.C. Cawley who provides the helpful SVM tool box. This work is supported in part by the National Natural Science Foundation of China under Grant No. 61673251, is also supported by the Key Science and

Technology Program of Shaanxi Province of China under Grant No. 2013K12-03-24, and is at the same time supported by the Fundamental Research Funds for the Central Universities under Grant No. GK201701006.

References

1. Abdi, M.J., Giveki, D.: Automatic detection of erythemato-squamous diseases using pso-svm based on association rules. Eng. Appl. Artif. Intell. **26**(1), 603–608 (2013)
2. Akay, M.F.: Support vector machines combined with feature selection for breast cancer diagnosis. Expert Syst. Appl. **36**(2), 3240–3247 (2009)
3. Bache, K., Lichman, M.: UCI machine learning repository (2013). http://archive.ics.uci.edu/ml
4. Blum, A., Langley, P.: Selection of relevant features and examples in machine learning. Artif. Intell. **97**(1–2), 245–271 (1997)
5. Chen, Y.W.: Combining svms with various feature selection strategies. Technical report Taiwan University (2005)
6. Fu, K.S., Min, P.J., Li, T.J.: Feature selection in pattern recognition. IEEE Trans. Syst. Sci. Cybern. **6**(1), 33–39 (1970)
7. Güvenir, H.A., Demiröz, G., İlter, N.: Learning differential diagnosis of erythemato-squamous diseases using voting feature intervals. Artif. Intell. Med. **13**(3), 147–165 (1998)
8. Güvenir, H.A., Emeksiz, N.: An expert system for the differential diagnosis of erythemato-squamous diseases. Expert Syst. Appl. **18**(1), 43–49 (2000)
9. Guyon, I., Elisseeff, A.: An introduction to variable and feature selection. JMLR **3**, 1157–1182 (2003)
10. Hua, J.P., Tembe, W.D., Dougherty, E.R.: Performance of feature-selection methods in the classification of high-dimension data. Pattern Recogn. **42**(3), 409–424 (2009)
11. Karabatak, M., Ince, M.C.: An expert system for detection of breast cancer based on association rules and neural network. Expert Syst. Appl. **36**(2), 3465–3469 (2009)
12. Karabatak, M., Ince, M.C.: A new feature selection method based on association rules for diagnosis of erythemato-squamous diseases. Expert Syst. Appl. **36**(10), 12500–12505 (2009)
13. Kohavi, R., John, G.H.: Wrappers for feature subset selection. Artif. Intell. **97**(1–2), 273–324 (1997)
14. Lin, T.Y.: Granular computing: From rough sets and neighborhood systems to information granulation and computing with words. In: European Congress on Intelligent Techniques and Soft Computing, pp. 1602–1606, September 8–12 1997
15. Liu, H.Q., Li, J.Y., Wong, L.: A comparative study on feature selection and classification methods using gene expression profiles and proteomic patterns. Genome Inf. **13**, 51–60 (2002)
16. Liu, H.W., Sun, J., Liu, L., Zhang, H.J.: Feature selection with dynamic mutual information. Pattern Recogn. **42**(7), 1330–1339 (2009)
17. Liu, Y., Zheng, Y.F.: Fs_sfs: a novel feature selection method for support vector machines. Pattern Recogn. **39**(7), 1333–1345 (2006)
18. Luukka, P.: Similarity classifier using similarity measure derived from yu's norms in classification of medical data sets. Comput. Biol. Med. **37**(8), 1133–1140 (2007)

19. Luukka, P., Leppälampi, T.: Similarity classifier with generalized mean applied to medical data. Comput. Biol. Med. **36**(9), 1026–1040 (2006)
20. Maio, D.Q., Wang, G.Y., Liu, Q.: Granular Computing: Past, Present and Prospects. China Science Press, Beijing (2007). in Chiniese
21. Marill, T., Green, D.M.: On the effectiveness of receptors in recognition systems. IEEE Trans. Inf. Theory **9**(1), 11–17 (1963)
22. Miranda, J., Montoya, R., Weber, R.: Linear penalization support vector machines for feature selection. In: Pal, S.K., Bandyopadhyay, S., Biswas, S. (eds.) PReMI 2005. LNCS, vol. 3776, pp. 188–192. Springer, Heidelberg (2005). doi:10.1007/11590316_24
23. Nanni, L.: An ensemble of classifiers for the diagnosis of erythemato-squamous diseases. Neurocomputing **69**(7), 842–845 (2006)
24. Özcift, A., Gülten, A.: Genetic algorithm wrapped bayesian network feature selection applied to differential diagnosis of erythemato-squamous diseases. Digit. Signal Proc. **23**(1), 230–237 (2013)
25. Polat, K., Günes, S.: The effect to diagnostic accuracy of decision tree classifier of fuzzy and k-nn based weighted pre-processing methods to diagnosis of erythemato-squamous diseases. Digit. Signal Proc. **16**(6), 992–930 (2006)
26. Polat, K., Günes, S.: A novel hybrid intelligent method based on c4.5 decision tree classifier and one-against-all approach for multi-class classification problems. Expert Syst. Appl. **36**(2), 1587–1592 (2009)
27. Übeyli, E.D.: Multiclass support vector machines for diagnosis of erythemato-squamous diseases. Expert Syst. Appl. **35**(8), 1733–1740 (2008)
28. Übeyli, E.D.: Combined neural networks for diagnosis of erythemato-squamous diseases. Expert Syst. Appl. **36**(3), 5107–5112 (2009)
29. Übeyli, E.D., Doğdu, E.: Automatic detection of erythemato-squamous diseases using k-means clustering. J. Med. Syst. **34**(2), 179–184 (2010)
30. Übeyli, E.D., Güler, I.: Automatic detection of erythemato-squamous diseases using adaptive neuro-fuzzy inference systems. Comput. Biol. Med. **35**(5), 421–433 (2005)
31. Vapnik, V.N.: The Nature of Statistical Learning Theory. Springer, New York (1995)
32. Wang, X.Y., Yang, J., Jensen, R., Liu, X.J.: Rough set feature selection and rule induction for prediction of malignancy degree in brain glioma. Comput. Methods Programs Biomed. **83**(2), 147–156 (2006)
33. Whitney, A.W.: A direct method of nonparametric measurement selection. IEEE Trans. Comput. **20**(9), 1100–1103 (1971)
34. Xie, J., Lei, J., Xie, W., Gao, X., Shi, Y., Liu, X.: Novel hybrid feature selection algorithms for diagnosing erythemato-squamous diseases. In: He, J., Liu, X., Krupinski, E.A., Xu, G. (eds.) HIS 2012. LNCS, vol. 7231, pp. 173–185. Springer, Heidelberg (2012). doi:10.1007/978-3-642-29361-0_21
35. Xie, J.Y., Lei, J.H., Xie, W.X., Shi, Y., Liu, X.H.: Two-stage hybrid feature selection algorithms for diagnosis of erythemato-squamous diseases. Health Inf. Sci. Syst. **1**(1), 1–10 (2013)
36. Xie, J.Y., Wang, C.X.: Using support vector machines with a novel hybrid feature selection method for diagnosis of erythemato-squamous diseases. Expert Syst. Appl. **38**(5), 5809–5815 (2011)

37. Xie, J.Y., Xie, W.X., Wang, C.X., Gao, X.B.: A novel hybrid feature selection method based on IFSFFS and SVM for the diagnosis of erythemato-squamous diseases. In: Diethe, T., Cristianini, N., Shawe-Taylor, J. (eds.) JMLR Workshop and Conference Proceedings, vol. 11: Workshop on Applications of Pattern Analysis, pp. 142–151. MIT press (2010)
38. Yao, Y.Y.: Granular computing for data mining. In: Dasarathy, B.V. (ed.) Proceedings of SPIE Conference on Data Mining, Intrusion Detection, Information Assurance, and Data Networks Security, pp. 1–12 (2006)
39. Zhang, Y., Xie, J.Y., Li, J., Chen, Y.Y., He, R.R., Li, Y.: Clustering analysis for erythemato-squamous diseases. J. Univ. Jinan Sci. Technol. **31**(3), 181–187 (2017)

A Semantically-Enabled System
for Inflammatory Bowel Diseases

Lei Xu[1(✉)], Zhisheng Huang[2], Hao Fan[1], and Siwei Yu[1]

[1] School of Information Management, Wuhan University, Wuhan, China
{xlei,hfan,manfisy}@whu.edu.cn
[2] Department of Computer Science, VU University Amsterdam,
Amsterdam, The Netherlands
huang@cs.vu.nl

Abstract. The incidence rate of Inflammatory Bowel Disease (IBD) in China is increasing in recent years and the cause of this disease is still not clear. In order to promote the development of this study, in this paper, we propose a Semantically-enabled System for Inflammatory Bowel Diseases (SeSIBD). It provides functions of semantic retrieval over patient data, statistical analysis and literature retrieval based on patient characteristics. SeSIBID is built on the top of LarKC, a semantic platform for scalable semantic data processing and reasoning. Although the current implementation of SeSIBID is a prototype system, it will provide an infrastructure for clinical decision making support for deep excavation and knowledge discovery on various of medical resources of IBD in the future.

Keywords: Inflammatory Bowel Diseases · Crohn's disease · Semantic technology · Semantic system

1 Introduction

Inflammtory Bowel Disease (IBD) includes Ulcerative Cllitis (UC) and Crohn's Disease (CD). It is a specific type of chronic intestinal inflammatory disease with unknown etiology and it is common in Europe and North America and other Western countries. Although the incidence rate in Asian countries is lower than in western countries, it is in the rapid growth, and the relevant epidemiological reports also become more and more [13]. The long-term follow-up on IBD patients is still lacking in China. As the IBD incidence rate increases in China, the epidemiological study becomes more urgent. With the epidemiological data, we may find possible causes, the characteristics of the diseases, and other important information for medical treatment. There are massive multi-source heterogeneous medical resources of IBD, including test and analysis data of basic medical research, medical literature, clinical diagnosis reports, patient medical records, medical image and a variety of medical database.

Thus, we need an effective knowledge organization method for data/knowledge integration of medical resources of IBD. The Semantic technology provides an

© Springer International Publishing AG 2017
S. Siuly et al. (Eds.): HIS 2017, LNCS 10594, pp. 69–80, 2017.
https://doi.org/10.1007/978-3-319-69182-4_8

effective approach for data integration, data sharing and reusability, and support for knowledge representation and reasoning [3,4,18]. It can meet this demand. In recent years, the semantic technology has been widely used in life science, biomedical domains and others.

In this paper, we propose a Semantically-enabled System for Inflammatory Bowel Diseases (SeSIBD). We have implemented a prototype of SeSIBD by using the semantic technology [3,4,7,18] to realize the basic functionalities for the medical data management, statistical analysis and medical literature retrieval for IBD. We have constructed the knowledge graphs of IBD for semantic queries and knowledge management. This work will provide the possibility for clinical decision making support. SeSIBID is built on the top of LarKC, a semantic platform for scalable semantic data processing and reasoning[1] [8]. In this paper we will report how SeSIBID can be implemented in LarKC and show some initial experiments with IBD patient data.

The rest of this paper is organized as follows: Sect. 2 proposes the architecture of Semantically-enabled system for IBD and discuss its implementation. Section 3 shows several semantic queries of SeSIBID. Section 4 presents the experiments of the system over a collection of patients of Crohn's disease in China. Section 6 discuss the future work, relevant work, before making the conclusions.

2   System

As we have discussed above, SeSIBD is built on the top of LarKC [8,23]. Which is a massive semantic data processing platform. Of course, SeSIBD can be built on other semantic platforms. The reason why we selected the LarKC platform is because it has the following distinguished features. In LarKC, different functions can be configured flexibly through plug-ins and this will realize functions control on the workflow level. The application program will call various plug-ins for different use through workflow. These plug-ins will get corresponding results through transformation, selection, reasoning and other operations on related data. There are five types of plug-ins in LarKC:

- Identifier plug-in: We use this type of plug-ins to obtain corresponding data according to search requirements. Data mining and machine learning technology also can be used to help data acquisition;
- Transformer plug-in: Data format can be changed by using these kinds of plug-ins;
- Selector plug-in: Using selector plug-ins, we can get a portion from big data, and this will make reasoning process more effective;
- Reasoner plug-in: Reasoner plug-ins provide various reasoning services, such as rule-based reasoning, inconsistent ontology reasoning, etc.
- Decider plug-in: According to the input and output data of plug-ins, decider plug-ins can make decision to realize functions control over workflow level.

---

[1] http://www.larkc.eu.

The architecture of SeSIBD is shown in Fig. 1. The Semantic data like IBD ontology, semantic patient data, PubMed dataset, and other biomedical ontologies or terminologies such as SNOMED CT and DrugBank can be loaded and managed by the data layer of LarKC. Meanwhile, the R-language, the statistical toolkit, will be used for statistical analysis over these data. Based on this work, we will carry out statistical analysis over massive medical semantic data and this work will be a great challenge; The core of LarKC provides APIs for data access and the returned data will be used by various plug-ins in the workflow to realize specific functions such as semantic queries, patient data and medical literature retrieval and so on. All functions are managed by the management module uniformly and deployed in Web servers with SPARQL endpoints. Here are the basic functions of SeSIBD:

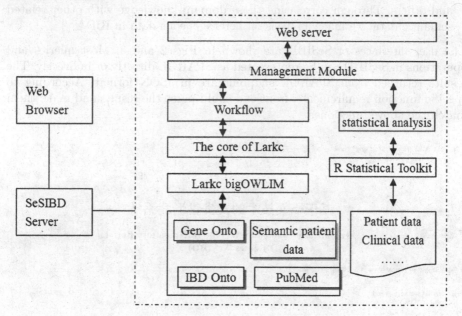

Fig. 1. Architecture of SeSIBD

- Semantic queries, namely SPARQL search. The user's query demands will be expressed in SPARQL and then sent to a SPARL endpoint.
- Patient data display. In the interface of this function, basic data, life mode data, diagnostic data and other data of patient can be shown.
- Statistical analysis. The IBD research involves many factors, such as patient's susceptibility, immune system, environmental factors and relationships between symbiotic microbes and hosts, and so on [15]. In this system, we use the R statistics package to realize the statistics analysis function, such as t test, factor analysis, principal component analysis, and so on, to discover potential relationships between these factors. At the same time, this paper is intended to study the statistical analysis on massive medical data.

- Literature retrieval. According to characteristics of patient data, literatures related to this patient's situation can be returned through semantic search over Linked Life Data[2]. Specifically, we can obtain some variables in this patient record and diagnosis a report combining with other related research results, such as specific genes or specific microbes associated with IBD. Using these data related to this patient, we construct SPARQL query statements to carry out semantic retrieval on PubMed semantic data. We could get relevant medical literatures for this patient's disease.
- Research analysis. We could find out data sources related to IBD such as gene, protein, microorganism through literature retrieval and domain experts. In this process, we construct a Knowledge Graphs of IBD, which consists of well-known biomedical ontologies/terminologies such as SNOMED CT, ICD10 and others. Through correlating those domain knowledge with other related semantic data, we make analysis on heterogeneous data in IBD.

The user interfaces of SeSIBD are shown in Figs. 2 and 3. Most queries and operations in SeSIBD can be represented as SPARQL directly or indirectly. The results returned from SPARQL endpoint are in JSON format. According to specific function requirements, front end could parse the results and make them match the above functions.

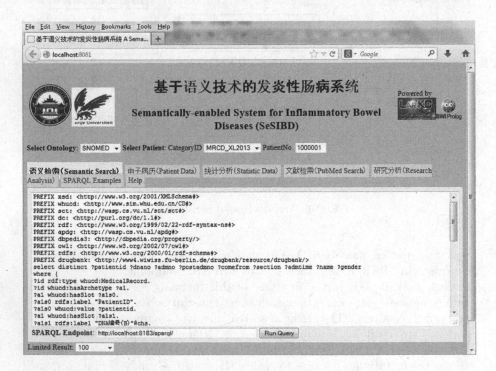

Fig. 2. Semantic search interface of SeSIBD

---

[2] http://linkedlifedata.com/.

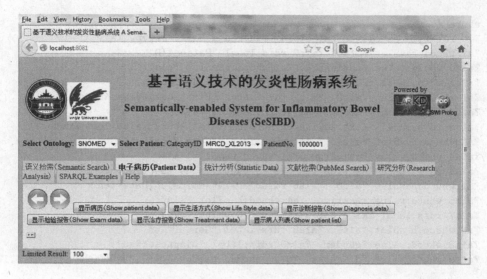

Fig. 3. Patient data interface of SeSIBD

3 Semantic Queries

In the following, we will show several concrete examples of semantic queries in the system.

Semantic Query 1: The patient data in SeSIBD is designed based on the idea of the archetype of medical records. We use the similar format of semantic patient data in APDG, a knowledge-based patient data generator[3]. The following SPARQL query shows a simple example how to obtain the DNA No. of a patient in that semantic patient data.

```
PREFIX ...
select distinct ?patientid ?dnano
where {
?id rdf:type whucd:MedicalRecord.
?id whucd:hasArchetype ?a1.
?a1 whucd:hasSlot ?a1s0. ?a1s0 rdfs:label "PatientID".
?a1s0 whucd:value ?patientid. ?a1 whucd:hasSlot ?a1s1.
?a1s1 rdfs:label "DNA No(B)"@en. ?a1s1 whucd:value ?dnano.
} LIMIT 300
```

Semantic Query 2: This semantic query shows how to search over more patient data with the values of patient ID, admission numbers and dates, patient name, gender, diagnose with the concept ID of Crohn's disease in the medical ontology SNOMED CT.

```
PREFIX ...
select distinct ?patientid ?dnano ?admno ?postadmno
  ?comefrom ?section ?admtime ?name ?gender
```

---
[3] http://wasp.cs.vu.nl/apdg.

```
where {
?id rdf:type whucd:MedicalRecord. ?id whucd:hasArchetype ?a1.
?a1 whucd:hasSlot ?a1s0. ?a1s0 rdfs:label "PatientID".
?a1s0 whucd:value ?patientid. ?a1 whucd:hasSlot ?a1s1.
?a1s1 rdfs:label "DNA No"@en. ?a1s1 whucd:value ?dnano.
?a1 whucd:hasSlot ?a1s2. ?a1s2 rdfs:label "First Admission No"@en.
?a1s2 whucd:value ?admno. ?a1 whucd:hasSlot ?a1s3.
?a1s3 rdfs:label "Next Admission No"@en. ?a1s3 whucd:value ?postadmno.
?a1 whucd:hasSlot ?a1s4. ?a1s4 rdfs:label "Come From"@en.
?a1s4 whucd:value ?comefrom. ?a1 whucd:hasSlot ?a1s5.
?a1s5 rdfs:label "Section"@en. ?a1s5 whucd:value ?section.
?a1 whucd:hasSlot ?a1s6. ?a1s6 rdfs:label "Admission Date"@en.
?a1s6 whucd:value ?admtime. ?a1 whucd:hasSlot ?a1s7.
?a1s7 rdfs:label "Name"@en. ?a1s7 whucd:value ?name.
?a1 whucd:hasSlot ?a1s8. ?a1s8 rdfs:label "Gender"@en.
?a1s8 whucd:value ?gender. ?a1s9 rdfs:label "Diagnose"@en.
?a1s9 whucd:value ?diagnose. ?a1s9 snomed:hasConceptID "34000006".
}
LIMIT 300
```

From the ontology of SNOMED CT, we have the following concept hierarchy (with their concept IDs) for IBD:

```
Inflammatory disorder of digestive system (disorder), Concept ID: 373407002
   Inflammatory disorder of digestive tractConcept ID: 128999004
      Inflammatory bowel disease, Concept ID: 24526004
         Crohn's disease (disorder), Concept ID: 34000006
            Arthritis co-occurrent and due to Crohn's disease (disorder),
                              Concept ID: 8161000119106
            Crohn disease of anal canal (disorder),Concept ID: 721702009
            Crohn's disease in remission, Concept ID: 426549001
            Crohn's stricture of colon, Concept ID: 413276006
            Gastrointestinal Crohn's disease (disorder),Concept ID: 397172008
            Iritis with Crohn's disease (disorder), Concept ID: 410485009
            Orofacial Crohn's disease (disorder), Concept ID: 196578009
            Perianal Crohn's disease, Concept ID: 235796008
```

If we want to search over patients who have the diagnosis as a special kind of Crohn's disease, i.e. Gastrointestinal Crohn's disease, the concept ID in the semantic query above can be replaced with the corresponding concept ID (for example, Concept ID:397172008) in the medical ontology.

4 Experiments

4.1 Basic Information

We have obtained a set of IBD patient data for the experiments with SeSIBD. Those dataset consists of 204 patients of Crohn's disease, which have been collected in Zhongnan Hospital of Wuhan City in China. According to other IBD studies and the rarity of this disease, the dataset of 204 cases is a large one already. This dataset contains the medical records from the year 1993 till the

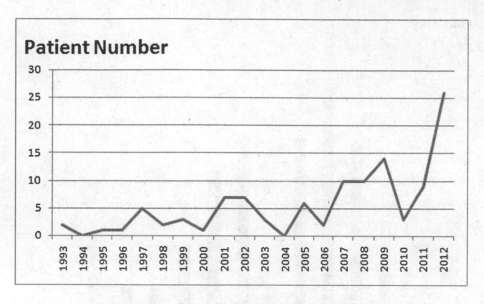

Fig. 4. Cases distribution of CD according to diagnosis year

year 2012. Of them, there are 111 patients with a diagnosis year. In Fig. 4, there is an increasing trend of IBD patients in recent years in Hubei province according to this dataset. This may due to the reputation of Zhongnan hospital of Wuhan University, which is famous for its research on IBD as a large 3A hospital in Hubei province, and IBD patients prefer to select this hospital for their treatments. It also may relate to other factors, for example, people's diet structure is increasingly westernized, patients can afford more expenses for medical examinations and treatments. There are 66 patients born after 1980's. Most patients come from big and middle cities (43 cases) and few patients come from village (9 cases) and small-town (8 cases). Most patients have discontinuous symptom of stomachache (125 cases). Most patients' early onset type is inflammatory (108 cases), and the number of penetrating type is 32, the number of constricting type is 48.

4.2   IBD Onset Distribution

Crohn's Disease (CD) has great onset rates in the adolescent and young adults, between 15 to 25 years old. A number of studies have discovered that the 2nd peak of incidence is between ages 50 to 80. CD is generally acknowledged to be more common in urban populations, but the work in this paper is conflicting on this point. As shown in Fig. 5, there are two peaks in the age distribution of CD, one is between 23 to 27 and another is between 38 to 42. Age and gender distribution of CD from different regions are shown in Fig. 6. In China, the mean age of onset with CD is about 10 years earlier than UC, just as that in Japan, Republic of Korea, and Western countries. But the peak age of the CD

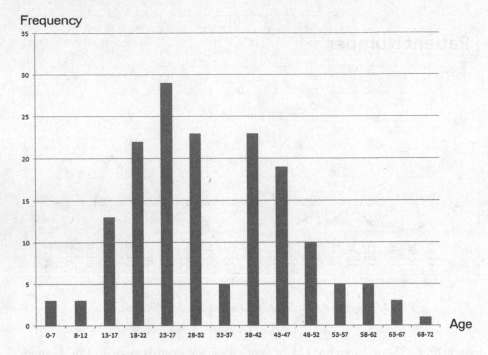

Fig. 5. Age distribution of CD

onset in Mainland China is older than that in other countries. Although Asian studies reported a similar peak age of onset for both UC and CD among Japan, Republic of Korea, and Western countries, the second smaller peak is more likely to occur in Western countries [22], with the exception of Japan, which has a second smaller peak age on 60?64 years old [14]. Latest study suggests a second smaller peak age on 45–54 years old in Hong Kong [6], but not found in Mainland China.

The average age of these patients is $33.22 + 12.69$. It is similar with the result in the study [26] in which the average age of patients is $33.3 + 14.76$. There are 121 male patients and 76 female patients (gender information of left cases is missed). The ratio between male and female patient is 1.59:1. This result is similar with that in the studies [1,2,5] in China. However, in west countries, the onset ratio between female and male is 1.1–1.8:1 [12,24], that means the number of female patients is a little higher than the number of male patients. That shows the difference between China and western countries. The biggest reason for this difference may be the differences of regional environment and ethnic genetics among these countries.

4.3   Season and Smoking Factors Analysis

Most patients came to see doctors between spring and summer seasons, this results is shown in Fig. 7, that means the time of the onset of CD is mainly at spring and summer. The same results can be found in [25]. In the figureref-fig:month, seasons are ranked according to the number of people in hospital.

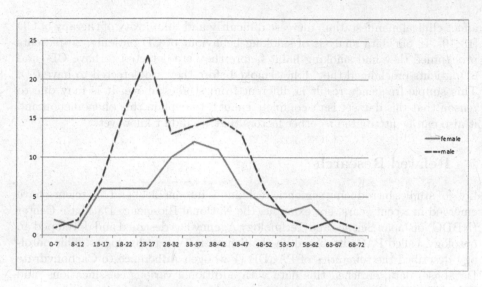

Fig. 6. Ages and gender distribution of CD

Summer is the season with the maximal number of patients. The next seasons are spring and autumn. It seems to suggest that IBD onset may be linked to the season change. Several studies agree that smoking is one of the pathogenesis of CD risk factors, and smoking can increase the CD risk. The condition will be even more complicated when comparing CD patients who have history of smoking with no smoking patients with CD [10]. Chinese case-control studies have shown that smoking may be a risk factor for CD [20]. The smoking can

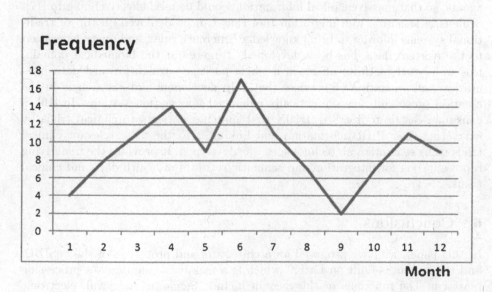

Fig. 7. Month distribution of CD

affect clinical manifestation, increase difficultly and complexity of therapy of CD [13,19]. In our data analysis of smoking behaviour of CD patients, 20 patients proclaimed they had smoking habit before they are detected to have CD, and 61 patients proclaimed they didn't smoke before they are detected to have CD. This simple frequency result is different from studies above. It is may due to reason that this dataset isn't complete enough to explain this phenomenon and it also can be attributed to other factors that we didn't know yet.

5   Related Research

Lots of studies introducing semantic techniques into medical and life science have emerged in recent years. For example, the National Bioscience Database Center (NBDC) of Japan Science and Technology Agency has designed and developed an ontology, called PAConto based on the Semantic Web technologies. This ontology described the semantics of PACDB (Pathogen Adherence to Carbohydrate Database) data, enriched this data with additional various classifications, and linked PACDB data with related biomedical resources. In addition, they have developed a system with a user interface, using which the users can retrieve and search information from PAConto [21]. In the study from [11], a ubiquitous smart hospital information system model under WaaS (Wisdom as a Service) architecture was proposed. And a smart medical knowledge recommendation system, namely SKeWa, was built to reveal the usefulness of the model and the methods. Union Hospital affiliated to Tongji School of Pharmacy of Huazhong University of Science and Technology introduced the advanced semantic technology into the monitoring on the use of antibacterial agents, innovatively put forward ideas to develop a semantically enabled system for rational use of antibacterial agents, so that massive clinical information would be used effectively [9]. In [17], Scaleus, a semantic web migration tool that can be deployed on top of traditional systems in order to bring knowledge, inference rules, and query federation to the existent data, has been developed. Targeted at the biomedical domain, this web-based platform offers, in a single package, straightforward data integration and semantic web services that help developers and researchers in the creation process of new semantically enhanced information systems. In [16], a consumer-centric tool called TrialX that matches patients to clinical trials by extracting their PHR information and linking it to the most relevant clinical trials using semantic web technologies was developed. It provides the underlying representation for integration and semantic retrieval of health data and clinical trials.

6   Conclusions

In this paper, we have proposed an architecture and prototype of the SeSIBD, and the system is built on LarKC which is a massive semantic data processing platform. The functions of this system include Semantic Retrieval, electronic medical record display, Statistical analysis, literature retrieval and Research analysis and so on. At present, the system is still in the early development stage and semantic analysis based on these data is also not deep enough, later we will make users' requirements clear and collaborate with experts in the IBD field to build semantic data foundation of IBD and improves the functions of this system.

We will continue to develop the system of SeSIBD by the integration with more biomedical ontologies such as UMLS, the gene ontology, the protein ontology UNIPROT, and others. We will make comprehensive analysis of the semantic patient data in the system with the support of the semantic technology to get more findings over the diseases. We will make the evaluation of the system by asking medical doctors to use it in realistic scenarios for clinical decision making. Based on structured medical knowledge graph and precise expression of query requirements, retrieval based on semantic web techniques have accurate results comparing to traditional retrieval methods which is based on lexical matching in most cases, but the usability assessment of this system is still needed to be carried out. We will leave them for future work.

Acknowledgments. This work was partially supported by a grant from the CSC (China Scholarship Council), the National Natural Science Foundation of China under grant number 71503189, the VU-China Cooperation fund, and the major cooperation project between mainland China and Taiwan under grant number 71661167007.

References

1. Al-Ghamdi, A.S., Al-Mofleh, I.A., Al-Rashed, R.S., Al-Amri, S.M., Aljebreen, A.M., Isnani, A.C., El-Badawi, R.: Epidemiology and outcome of crohn's disease in a teaching hospital in Riyadh. World J. Gastroenterol. **10**(9), 1341–1344 (2004)
2. Chinese IBD APDW2004: Retrospective analysis of 515 cases of crohns disease hospitalization in China: nationwide study from 1990 to 2003. J. Gastroenterol. Hepatol. **21**, 1009–1015 (2006)
3. Berners-Lee, T.: The semantic web. Sci. Am. **284**, 28–37 (2001)
4. Berners-Lee, T., Hendler, J., Lassila, O.: The semantic web. Sci. Am. Mag. **284**, 34–43 (2001)
5. Chow, D.K., Leong, R.W., Lai, L.H., Wong, G.L., Leung, W.-K., Chan, F.K., Sung, J.J.: Changes in crohn's disease phenotype over time in the chinese population: validation of the montreal classification system. Inflammatory Bowel Dis. **14**(4), 536–541 (2008)
6. Chow, D.K., Leong, R.W., Tsoi, K.K., Ng, S.S., Leung, W.-K., Wu, J.C., Wong, V.W., Chan, F.K., Sung, J.J.: Long-term follow-up of ulcerative colitis in the Chinese population. Am. J. Gastroenterol. **104**(3), 647–654 (2009)
7. Feigenbaum, L.: The semantic web in action. Sci. Am. **297**, 90–97 (2007)
8. Fensel, D., van Harmelen, F., Andersson, B., Brennan, P., Cunningham, H., Della Valle, E., Fischer, F., Huang, Z., Kiryakov, A., Lee, T., School, L., Tresp, V., Wesner, S., Witbrock, M., Zhong, N.: Towards LarKC: a platform for web-scale reasoning. In: Proceedings of the IEEE International Conference on Semantic Computing (ICSC 2008). IEEE Computer Society Press, CA, USA (2008)
9. Hua, X., Chen, C., Huang, Z., Hu, Q., Gu, J., Yu, S., Chen, D.: Intelligent monitoring on use of antibacterial agents based on semantic technology. China Digital Med. 4:006 (2013)

10. Kennelly, R.P., Subramaniam, T., Egan, L.J., Joyce, M., et al.: Smoking and crohn's disease: active modification of an independent risk factor (education alone is not enough). J. Crohn's Colitis **7**(8), 631–35 (2013)

11. Li, Y., Wan, Z., Huang, J., Chen, J., Huang, Z., Zhong, N.: A smart hospital information system for mental disorders. In: 2015 IEEE/WIC/ACM International Conference on Web Intelligence and Intelligent Agent Technology (WI-IAT), vol. 1, pp. 321–324. IEEE (2015)

12. Loftus, C.G., Loftus, E.V., Harmsen, W.S., Zinsmeister, A.R., Tremaine, W.J., Melton, L.J., Sandborn, W.J.: Update on the incidence and prevalence of crohn's disease and ulcerative colitis in olmsted county, minnesota, 1940–2000. Inflammatory Bowel Dis. **13**(3), 254–261 (2007)

13. Min, L.: The changing profiles of inflammatory bowel disease in china-a 15 year review of IBD cases to a large hospital in eastern China. Technical report (2011)

14. Oriuchi, T., Hiwatashi, N., Kinouchi, Y., Takahashi, S., Takagi, S., Negoro, K., Shimosegawa, T.: Clinical course and longterm prognosis of Japanese patients with crohns disease: predictive factors, rates of operation, and mortality. J. Gastroenterol. **38**(10), 942–953 (2003)

15. Ouyang, Q., Wang, Y., Hu, R.: Epidemiology of inflammatory bowel disease in China. Chinese J. Digestion **28**(12), 814–818 (2008)

16. Patel, C., Gomadam, K., Khan, S., Garg, V.: Trialx: using semantic technologies to match patients to relevant clinical trials based on their personal health records. J. Web Sem. **8**(4), 342–347 (2010)

17. Sernadela, P., González-Castro, L., Oliveira, J.L.: Scaleus: semantic web services integration for biomedical applications. J. Med. Syst. **41**(4), 54 (2017)

18. Shadbolt, N., Hall, W., Berners-Lee, T.: The semantic web revisited. IEEE Intell. Syst. **21**, 96–101 (2006)

19. Shanwen, C., Pengyuan, W. Yunchun, L., et al.: Research progress on risk factors associated with postoperative recurrence in patients with Crohn's disease after bowel resection (1), 89–92 (2015)

20. X. Shi, J. Zheng, Z. Guo, F. Chen, and Z. Wang. Correlated pathogenetic factors of crohn's disease: a case-control study **13**(5), 293–296 (2008)

21. Solovieva, E., Fujita, N., Shikanai, T., Aoki-Kinoshita, K.F., Narimatsu, H.: PAConto: RDF representation of PACDB data and ontology of infectious diseases known to be related to glycan binding. In: Aoki-Kinoshita, K.F. (ed.) A Practical Guide to Using Glycomics Databases, pp. 261–295. Springer, Tokyo (2017). doi:10.1007/978-4-431-56454-6_14

22. Thia, K.T., Loftus, E.V., Sandborn, W.J., Yang, S.-K.: An update on the epidemiology of inflammatory bowel disease in Asia. Am. J. Gastroenterol. **103**(12), 3167–3182 (2008)

23. Witbrock, M., Fortuna, B., Bradesko, L., Kerrigan, M., Bishop, B., van Harmelen, F., ten Teije, A., Oren, E., Momtchev, V., Tenschert, A., Cheptsov, A., Roller, S., Gallizo, G.: D5.3.1 - requirements analysis and report on lessons learned during prototyping. Larkc project deliverable, June 2009

24. Yang, G., Guo, B., Lu, W., et al.: Document analysis on the misdiagnosis of Crohns disease. Chin. J. Misdiagn. **7**(21), 5015–5026 (2007)

25. Ying, Z.: Case analysis of Crohn's disease in the first classified 3A hospital in Jilin. (1), 89–92 (2016)

26. Zheng, J.J., Zhu, X.S., Huangfu, Z., Shi, X.H., Guo, Z.R.: Prevalence and incidence rates of crohn's disease in mainland China: a meta-analysis of 55 years of research. J. Dig. Dis. **11**(3), 161–166 (2010)

Early Classification of Multivariate Time Series Based on Piecewise Aggregate Approximation

ChaoHong Ma[✉], XiaoQing Weng, and ZhongNan Shan

Information Technology College, Hebei University of Economics & Business,
Shijiazhuang 050061, China
chaohma@126.com

Abstract. Early Classification on Time Series is becoming more significant in the field of Time Series Data Ming. Especially in some time-sensitive filed, it is obviously preferred to make earlier classification, such as Medical science, Health informatics et al. However, the research tasks are mainly focused on UTS, those of MTS are less. MTS is faced with variable-based and time-based dimensionality. It is significant to find appropriate dimensionality reduction in the practical application of early classification on multivariate time series. We propose a novel method MTEECP based on center sequence and Piecewise Aggregate Approximation which achieve early classification in low-dimension space. Experimental results on 6 real datasets intuitively show our proposed method can reach favorable early classification on MTS.

Keywords: Early classification · Center sequence · Multivariate time series · Piecewise aggregate approximation

1 Introduction

Any kind of real-value sequences in order can be seen as time series [1], so time series classification is of great use, such as medical diagnosis, disaster prediction et al. Also, earlier classification [2] is favorable for decision in some time-sensitive domain.

Nowadays, the research of Early classification mainly focus on univariate time series (UTS), such as ECTS [2, 9], RelClass [3], EDSC [4], ECDIRE [5].

Multivariate time series (MTS) is also universal in real life [6], for example, the daily records of a patient may contain temperature, blood pressure, pulse and other factors. The less research of Early Classification on Multivariate Time Series (ECMTS) is due to the following factors:

a. MTS have the curse of dimensionality. *b*. It is much complicated relationship among variables. *c*. The number of variables is large and redundancy existed.

Those lead to lees research of MTS and the early classification methods on UTS can't directly apply on MTS. Now the MTS is increasing in various fields, so the research on the Early Classification of MTS is of theoretical and practical significance.

The dimensionality reduction [7] of MTS data can be divided into two aspects, variable-based and time-based dimension. One is the number of variables, another is

S. Siuly et al. (Eds.): HIS 2017, LNCS 10594, pp. 81–88, 2017.
https://doi.org/10.1007/978-3-319-69182-4_9

the length of MTS data. As the specialization of early classification and the properties of MTS, most of the methods failed to utilize in the practical application of ECMTS.

Previous studies on ECMTS mainly focus on extracting shapelets, explainable features which in a sense can represent the characteristic of one class. All these faced large calculation, and didn't consider the relationship among variables.

In this paper, we proposed a novel strategy for ECMTS which combine center sequence [7] and Piecewise Aggregate Approximation [8] (PAA) into ECMTS. Our method solves the bottleneck that methods on UTS can't be applied in MTS, and reduced the computational complexity. Experimental results on real datasets show our method can effectively achieve better accuracy and earliness.

The structure of this paper is organized as follows. Section 2 gives the definitions and background in this paper. In Sect. 3, we review the related work. We propose our method MTSECP in Sect. 4. We present the experiment results In Sect. 5. Finally, we conclude this paper and future work in Sect. 6.

2   Background

Definition 1 Time Series. $X = [X_1, X_2, ..., X_k, X_m]$, $(m \geq 2)$, is a Multivariate Time Series, m denotes the number of variables, and k represents k-th variable. Each component X_k is a n-length Univariate Time Series. When $m = 1$, $t = X_1 = \{x_1, x_2, ..., x_n\}$, $x_i(1 \leq i \leq n)$ denotes the value in time i, n is the full length of time series t.

Definition 2 Center Sequence. Suppose X is a MTS, the center sequence [3] of MTS X we denoted by X', k stands for k-th variable, X'_i X'_i is the numerical value of center-sequence X' in time i. As follows, note that X' is a UTS.

$$X' = mean(X) = \frac{1}{m} \sum_{k=1}^{m} X_k \tag{1}$$

$$X'_i = \frac{\sum_{k=1}^{m} x_{ki}}{m} \tag{2}$$

Definition 3 Reverse Nearest Neighbors. Let t $(1, l)$ is the prefix of UTS t in time l, and in the space of prefix R^l, the Reverse Nearest Neighbors [2] of t is denoted by $RNN^l(t)$. $RNN^l(t) = \{t' \in T| t \in NN^l(t')\}$, thus if t is the nearest neighbor of t', we call t' is the reverse nearest neighbor of t. t and t' are all the samples of dataset *PCTRAIN* after the process of center sequence & PAA. $NN^l(t')$ is the set of the nearest neighbor for t'.

Definition 4 Minimum Prediction Length. Minimum Prediction Length [2] of t is defined by $MPL(t)$, as $MPL(t) = h$, if and only if for arbitrary l $(h < l < n)$ meets the follow conditions:
a. $RNN^l(t) = RNN^n(t) \neq \phi$; b. $RNN^{h-1}(t) \neq RNN^n(t)$. Specially, when $RNN^n(t) = \phi$, $MPL(t) = n$.

Definition 5 MPLs of Cluster. The MPLs of cluster S, $MPL(S)$ for short [2], where S is a cluster, when $MPL(S) = h$, if and only if for any l ($h < l < n$), satisfy the following limits: a. $RNN^l(S) = RNN^n(S)$; b. In prefix space R^l, S is 1NN consistent; c. when $l = h - 1$, limits a. and b. can't be satisfied.

Definition 6 Accuracy. Accuracy is the probability of true class results when test on test set, where $\hat{C}_i$ is the actual class label of the i-th test sample, C_i is the class label given by classifier, N is the sample number of $TEST$. $I(\cdot)$ is a function which equal to 1 when the equation within parentheses is true, otherwise 0.

$$Accurancy = \frac{1}{N} \sum_{i=1}^{N} I(\hat{C}_i = C_i) \tag{3}$$

Definition 7 Earliness. Earliness is evaluated by the length of time series used in early classification. We use the percentage as follow, where t_i is the i-th sample in $TEST$ data set.

$$Earliness = \frac{1}{N} \sum_{i=1}^{N} \frac{length(t_i)}{n} \times 100 \tag{4}$$

PAA is a common dimensionality reduction method. Firstly, divide the series into equal length segments, then calculate the mean of each segment, replace the numeric value of segment with its mean. PAA is of linear complexity and implement simply which is suitable for time series in the practical application of early classification.

Suppose that $t = X_1 = \{x_1, x_2, \ldots, x_i, \ldots, x_n\}$, $\overline{X_1}$ is the PAA representation of X_1, where n is the length of t, d is the number of segments we divided.

$$\overline{X_1} = \{\overline{x_1}, \ldots, \overline{x_i}, \ldots, \overline{x_d}\} \tag{5}$$

$$\overline{x_i} = \frac{d}{n} \sum_{j=\frac{n}{d}(i-1)+1}^{\frac{n_i}{d}} x_j \tag{6}$$

3 Related Work

Xing et al. [2, 9] applied 1-Nearest-Neighbor classifier to early classification on UTS, and proposed Early Classification on Time Series (ECTS).

Ghalwash et al. proposed a feature-based method, Multivariate Shapelets Detection [10] (MSD) extract multivariate shapelets composed of multiple segments. The segments in a MTS are of same begin and end point. He et al. [11, 12] present Mining Core Feature for Early Classification (MCFEC) which extracts shapelet candidates for every variable of MTS data independently which the candidates set is extremely large, and the begin and end point need not to be same. Lin et al. [13] present a reliable Early Classification on MTS with numerical and categorical attributes called REACT.

The above related works exist the following problems:

a. MSD and MCFEC all of high computational complexity.
b. Most of methods didn't consider the relationship among variables.
c. Shapelets extracted by MSD can't cover total distinctive patterns unless the length of shapelet is long enough. For MCFEC, because of the noise, some variables can match shapelets, but others can't, yet different variable may match different shapelet.

Faced with above problems, we propose Multivariate Time Series Early Classification based on PAA (MTSECP), combine center sequence with PAA to achieve early classification, and avoid issues caused by the shapelets and improve the performance.

4   Multivariate Time Series Early Classification Based on PAA

We present MTSECP which first use center sequence to get the UTS presentation of MTS, then apply PAA on center sequence, finally, execute early classification on PAA representation dataset. The program of MTSECP is shown in Algorithm 1.

Algorithm 1. MTSECP

Input: MTS train set *TRAIN*, MTS test set *TEST*, PAA dimensionality d
output: Accuracy, Earliness

1: For every MTS sample X ($m*n$) in *TRAIN*, calculate the center-sequence of X as one-dimensional representation X' ($1*n$), all the X' constitute new train set *CTRAIN*.

2: For every $X' \in CTRAIN$, divide X' into d segments with equal length $l_p = \frac{n}{d}$, then compute the mean of each segment

3: Take the means of d segments as the representation of X' denoted by X_p', the new dataset called *PCTRAIN*

4: In all prefix space R^l ($1 \leq l \leq n$), find the nearest neighbor of all the objects of *PCTRAIN*

5: Use single link multi-level hierarchical clustering to cluster *PCTRAIN*, get several clusters S

6: Calculate the MPLs of every leaf clusters, and assign $MPL(S)$ to every object in S

7: Iterate to get the nearest cluster pair (S_1, S_2), during each iteration integrate S_1 and S_2 into one parent cluster

8: For $X_p' \in S$, when $MPL(X_p') < MPL(S)$, assign $MPL(S)$ to $MPL(X_p')$

9: When all $X_p' \in S$, $MPL(X_p') \leq MPL(S)$, iteration stop

10: For every $Y \in TEST$, in time i ($1 \leq i \leq n$), $Y_i' = \frac{1}{m}\sum_{k=1}^{m} Y_k$, thus we obtain the MTS center-sequence representation before i, according to l_p in step 2, get PAA representation center-sequence Y_p'

11: At time i, if the nearest neighbor of Y_p' i.e. $NN_i(Y_p')$, the $MPL(NN_i(Y_p')) = i$, return the class label of $NN_i(Y_p')$ as the label of Y

12: If at time i, didn't exist the $NN_i(Y_p')$ like last step 11, we state classifier can't make reliable, then wait for more sequence of Y

13: Calculate the *accuracy* and *earliness*

MTSECP has three stages. Step 1–3 is dimensionality reduction phase, center-sequence and PAA both are of linear complexity, the cost is $O(m * n)$, m denotes the number of variables, n is the length of series, in general, m is much less than n ($m << n$). Step 4–9 is training stage, cluster data with multi-level hierarchical clustering [14] in all prefix space, then compute similarities between samples, time cost [2] is $O(|TR|^3 \cdot n)$, $|TR|$ is the number of train set. Thirdly, early classification is step 10–13, find the nearest neighbor of test set in train set, time cost is $O(|TE| \cdot n)$, where $|TE|$ is the number of test set. So the total complexity of MTSECP is $O(m * n + |TR|^3 \cdot n + |TE| \cdot n)$.

5 Experiment

We experimentally examine the performance of MTSECP. We implement MTSECP on 6 MTS datasets. All experiments are of 10-fold cross-validation scheme.

5.1 Dataset

The brief descriptions of the datasets we used in experiment are as follows.

BCI [16, 17] contains 2 classes, one is the electroencephalogram use left hand fingers to press keyboard, one is those use right hand fingers. Every MTS has 28 variables.

Wafer [18, 19] has 2 classes, normal and abnormal. In the semiconductor factory, each wafer can be described as a MTS with 6 variables.

ECG dataset [18, 19] contains 2 classes, normal and abnormal, use 2 electric poles to collect Electrocardiogram data in one single beat of heart. Each MTS has 2 variables.

Character Trajectories [15] is the pen tip trajectories, has 20 classes. All objects come from the same person, and record 3-dimention.

Lp1 and Lp4 datasets are robot execution failures [15]. Lp1 has 4 classes, Lp4 has 3. Every sample is 6-variable MTS. Table 1 shows the summary of the datasets.

Table 1. Summary of datasets used in experiments

Dataset	Num of variables	Max length	Min length	Num of labels	Num of samples
BCI	28	500	500	2	416
Wafer	6	198	104	2	327
ECG	2	152	39	2	200
Character Trajectories	3	205	109	20	2858
Lp1	6	15	15	4	88
Lp4	6	15	15	3	117

5.2 Experiment Results

This section, we use CSEC as the baseline which only use center sequence representation of MTS to call ECTS. The experiment results are shown in Table 2.

Table 2. Results using baseline method and MTSECP.

Dataset	CSEC		MTSECP	
	Accu	Earl	Accu	Earl
Wafer	88.97	59.29	97.56	57.35
BCI	52.29	94.05	69.64	93.88
ECG	85.42	61.00	94.39	53.83
Character Trajectories	95.66	69.90	96.72	69.54
Lp1	54.63	82.42	71.94	73.81
Lp4	56.31	91.86	71.06	67.42
Average	72.21	76.42	83.55	69.31

Table 2 shows the result. The Wilcoxon signed ranks test of accuracy and earliness between CSEC and MTSECP are both 0.03, 0.03 which revealed that MTSECP can get better results.

MTSECP can improve the performance of early classifier. May because PAA reduced dimensionality, smooth noise and reduce the deviation of outliers.

5.3 Parameter Analysis

MTSECP has a parameter d, PAA dimensionality stands for the number of segments the series divided. The range of d is from 2 to n, n is the length of series, choose the optimal d using in subsequent early classification phase. Figures 1 and 2 shows the results, horizontal axis is accuracy and earliness, vertical is PAA dimensionality d.

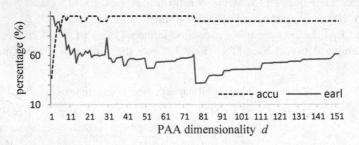

Fig. 1. The accuracy and earliness vs. PAA dimensionality on ECG dataset.

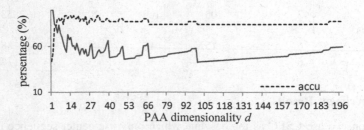

Fig. 2. The accuracy and earliness vs. PAA dimensionality on Wafer dataset.

Figures 1 and 2 are respectively the accuracy and earliness on Wafer, ECG. The accuracy begin to grows, then tends to be stable. The tendency in earliness is declining though have fluctuations. MTSECP can get preferable accuracy as earlier as possible.

6   Conclusion and Future Work

We proposed MTSECP, and results show MTSECP can apply in real dataset for early classification. Next, we plan to combine feature subset selection with MTSECP.

References

1. Yuan, J.D., Wang, Z.-H.: Review of time series representation and classification techniques. Comput. Sci. **42**(3), 1–7 (2015)
2. Xing, Z., Pei, J., Yu, P.S.: Early prediction on time series: a nearest neighbor approach. In: Proceedings of the International Joint Conference on Artificial Intelligence (IJCAI 2009), Pasadena, pp. 1297–1302, July 2009
3. Parrish, N., Anderson, H.S., Gupta, M.R., et al.: Classifying with confidence from incomplete information. J. Mach. Learn. Res. **14**(1), 3561–3589 (2013)
4. Xing, Z., Pei, J., Yu, P.S., et al.: Extracting interpretable features for early classification on time series. In: Eleventh SIAM International Conference on Data Mining (SDM 2011), 28–30 April 2011, Mesa, pp. 744–757 (2011)
5. Mori, U., Mendiburu, A., Keogh, E., et al.: Reliable early classification of time series based on discriminating the classes over time. Data Min. Knowl. Disc. **31**(1), 1–31 (2017)
6. Weng, X., Shen, J.: Classification of multivariate time series using two-dimensional singular value decomposition. Knowl. Based Syst. **21**(7), 535–539 (2008)
7. Li, H.: Piecewise aggregate representations and lower-bound distance functions for multivariate time series. Phys. A Stat. Mech. Appl. **427**, 10–25 (2015)
8. Keogh, E., Chakrabarti, K., Pazzani, M., et al.: Dimensionality reduction for fast similarity search in large time series databases. Knowl. Inf. Syst. **3**(3), 263–286 (2001)
9. Xing, Z., Pei, J., Yu, P.S.: Early classification on time series. Knowl. Inf. Syst. **31**(1), 105–127 (2012)
10. Ghalwash, M.F., Obradovic, Z.: Early classification of multivariate temporal observations by extraction of interpretable shapelets. BMC Bioinform. **13**(1), 1–12 (2012)
11. He, G., Duan, Y., Zhou, G., Wang, L.: Early classification on multivariate time series with core features. In: Decker, H., Lhotská, L., Link, S., Spies, M., Wagner, Roland R. (eds.) DEXA 2014. LNCS, vol. 8644, pp. 410–422. Springer, Cham (2014). doi:10.1007/978-3-319-10073-9_35
12. He, G., Duan, Y., Peng, R., et al.: Early classification on multivariate time series. Neurocomputing **149**(PB), 777–787 (2015)
13. Lin, Y.-F., Chen, H.-H., Tseng, V.S., Pei, J.: Reliable early classification on multivariate time series with numerical and categorical attributes. In: Cao, T., Lim, E.-P., Zhou, Z.-H., Ho, T.-B., Cheung, D., Motoda, H. (eds.) PAKDD 2015. LNCS, vol. 9077, pp. 199–211. Springer, Cham (2015). doi:10.1007/978-3-319-18038-0_16
14. Ding, C., He, X.: Cluster aggregate inequality and multi-level hierarchical clustering. In: Jorge, A.M., Torgo, L., Brazdil, P., Camacho, R., Gama, J. (eds.) PKDD 2005. LNCS, vol. 3721, pp. 71–83. Springer, Heidelberg (2005). doi:10.1007/11564126_12

15. Lichman, M.: UCI Machine Learning Repository. University of California, School of Information and Computer Science, Irvine (2013). http://archive.ics.uci.edu/ml
16. Blankertz, B., Curio, G., Müller, K.R.: Classifying single trial EEG: towards brain computer interfacing. In: Proceedings of the 2001 Neural Information Processing Systems (NIPS) Conference, pp. 157–164 (2001)
17. http://ida.first.fhg.de/projects/bci/competition_ii/
18. Olszewski, R.T.: Generalized Feature Extraction for Structural Pattern Recognition in Time-Series Data. Carnegie Mellon University, Pittsburgh (2001)
19. http://www.cs.cmu.edu/~bobski/

A Data-Driven Approach for Discovering the Recent Research Status of Diabetes in China

Xieling Chen[1], Heng Weng[2(✉)], and Tianyong Hao[3(✉)]

[1] School of Economics, Jinan University, Guangzhou, China
shaylyn_chen@163.com
[2] The Second Affiliated Hospital of Guangzhou University of Chinese Medicine,
Guangzhou, China
ww128@qq.com
[3] School of Information Science and Technology,
Guangdong University of Foreign Studies, Guangzhou, China
haoty@gdufs.edu.cn

Abstract. This paper aims at discovering the recent research status of diabetes in China through a data-driven bibliometrics and knowledge mapping analysis method on diabetes-related literature. With the basis of 24,561 publication documents from CNKI during 2007–2016, the quantitative analysis are conducted in three aspects: (1) descriptive statistical method for acquiring literature distribution characteristics; (2) hierarchical clustering, k-means clustering analysis, and multidimensional scaling analysis based on a keyword co-occurrence matrix for discovering research hotspots; and (3) network analysis for revealing cooperation relationships among authors and affiliations. The result shows some findings about the recent diabetes research in China. It also demonstrates the close cooperation of diabetes research among productive authors and affiliations through network generation and visualization.

Keywords: Diabetes · Distribution characteristics · Research hotspots · Cooperation network

1 Introduction

Diabetes and its complications are now the major health killers in most countries. According to International Diabetes Federation [1], 415 million or 8.8% of adults aged 20–79 had diabetes in 2015. The number is estimated to be 642 million in 2040. Not only does diabetes pose great threat to worldwide health, but it makes substantial economic impact on countries and national health systems. China is the top 1 country with the most people suffering from diabetes. According to Chinese Diabetes Society [2], there were nearly 110 million people with diabetes in China in 2014 with the overall prevalence doubling to 9.7% in nearly 10 years. The number of people at high risk was 150 million with the prevalence of pre-diabetes up to 15.5%, which was higher than the world average. Compared with the worldwide situation, threaten brought by diabetes is more severe in China.

© Springer International Publishing AG 2017
S. Siuly et al. (Eds.): HIS 2017, LNCS 10594, pp. 89–101, 2017.
https://doi.org/10.1007/978-3-319-69182-4_10

The research of diabetes has been always of an extensive concern in academia. Doctors and researchers have published a wealth of diabetes literatures to record their clinical and research findings. These research literatures can to some extent reflect the development of diabetes prevention and treatment. However, it is difficult to accurately capture the pulse through traditional manual retrieval when facing with diabetes literatures of such a large quantity, wide distribution and fast growth. Therefore, it is of need to develop an automatic, efficient, and accurate method to continuously discover the recent research status of diabetes.

Bibliometrics uses relevant statistical and mathematical approaches to study information materials, which has become a well-established part of information research to the quantitative description of documents [3]. Traditional bibliometrics is popular in solving problems of extreme value and sorting, but it is weak in revealing the structure of literature, e.g., the cooperation among authors and affiliations, the structure and evolution of research hotspots. On the other hand, knowledge mapping analysis is a widely applied graphical and visual technique in revealing structure relationship and scientific knowledge development process [4]. Technologies involving in mathematics, information science, and computer science are combined to help analyze and understand the development process and forefront issues [5]. To a certain extent, knowledge mapping analysis and bibliometrics can be regarded as complements for each other.

This paper presents a data-driven method based on bibliometrics and knowledge mapping analysis, aiming at discovering the recent research status of diabetes in China. Using the techniques of descriptive statistics, clustering and multidimensional scaling, and network analysis, this paper conducts the analysis on literature distribution characteristics, research hotspots and cooperation relationships. We believe that the work can potentially assist clinical professionals and medical researchers in determining hot research topics and keeping abreast of the research status of diabetes in the development of research strategies.

2   Literature Review

There have been a considerable number of studies with the applications of bibliometrics and knowledge mapping analysis: evaluate the speed of publication of ophthalmology journals [6], map the literature related to a certain research field such as cancer research [7, 8] or health literacy research [9], and allow one to recognize new topics in the literature [10]. Bibliometrics and knowledge mapping analysis have played fundamental roles in examining the trends in medical research output. Ramos [11] conducted a bibliometric analysis of tuberculosis research indexed in PubMed during 1997 and 2006, finding the phenomenon that the research output in countries with more estimated cases of tuberculosis was less than that in industrialized countries. Boudry et al. [12] provided a review on scientific production related with the field of eye disease during 2010 and 2014 so as to identify the major topics as well as the predominant actors including journals, countries, and continents. Similar works have been conducted for other medical fields, such as obesity [13], leishmaniasis [14], methaemoglobinaemia [15], giardiasis [16], dermatology [17], neurogenic bladder [18], rheumatology [19], and surgery [20].

Few studies concerning with diabetes using bibliometrics and knowledge mapping analysis methods can be found. Harande [21] used bibliometric approach to examine the increasing diabetes-related literature in Nigeria, indicating that the literature of diabetes in Nigeria was in harmony with the Bradford–Zipf distribution. Harande and Alhaji [22] examined the growth of published literature on the disease in three countries including Nigeria, Argentina and Thailand, showing that the literature of diabetes grew and spread very widely. Similar research has been done for diabetes literature in Middle East countries [23]. Geaney et al. [24] provided a detailed evaluation of type 2 diabetes mellitus research output during 1951–2012 with methods of large-scale data analysis, bibliometric indicators, and density-equalizing mapping. Zhang et al. [25] investigated the relationship between antipsychotics and type 2 diabetes research with bibliometrics method. The existing relative studies seldom focus on the literature of diabetes in China, let alone use the combination methods of bibliometrics and knowledge mapping analysis.

Therefore, the aim of this study is to provide a detailed evaluation of the diabetes research output from 2007 to 2016 in China using a data-driven method based on bibliometrics and knowledge mapping analysis to quantitatively analyze data from the CNKI database in terms of: (1) literature distribution characteristics with method of descriptive statistics; (2) research hotspots with method of clustering and multidimensional scaling analysis; and (3) cooperation relationships among authors and affiliations with network analysis methods.

3 The Data-Driven Approach

With the combination of bibliometrics and knowledge mapping analysis, we design a data-driven approach for discovering the recent research status of diabetes in mainland China from medical literature. The processing procedure is shown as Fig. 1. Diabetes-related publications as raw data are retrieved from CNKI and are used as dataset after preprocessing for bibliometrics and knowledge mapping analysis. The analysis applies descriptive statistical methods for acquiring literature distribution characteristics, multidimensional scaling analysis and data mining methods such as k-means clustering for discovering research hotspots, as well as network analysis for revealing cooperation relationships among authors and affiliations. Specifically, the procedure can be divided into the following stages:

Literature retrieval: The relevant publications were directly retrieved from CNKI in April 2017 with the following searching criteria: (1) "diabetes" as topic using an extended search keyword list; (2) "2007" to "2016" as publication year; (3) SCI, EI, CSSCI, and core journals as literature sources to keep high literature quality. The total retrieved raw data containing 35,059 documents was obtained for preprocessing.

Data preprocessing: to make sure of the high relevance with diabetes research, further data cleaning and processing was needed, consisting of: (1) excluding articles belonging to messaging literature like yearbooks, newspapers, and non-academic book publications; (2) excluding articles whose titles and keywords did not contain high

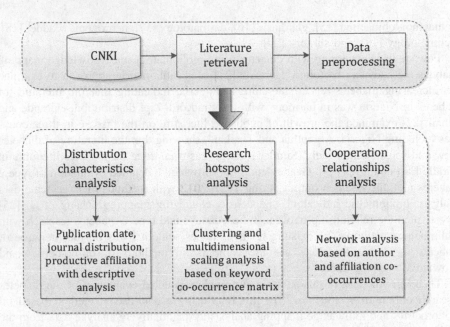

Fig. 1. The procedure for acquiring research status of diabetes in China

relevant words like "diabetes" and "hypoglycemic"; (3) keeping all the articles whose source journal names contained the keyword "diabetes". After preprocessing, we finally acquired the dataset containing 24,561 articles.

Distribution characteristics analysis: with the basis of 24,561 documents, the literature distribution characteristics including publication date and journal distribution as well as productive affiliations were acquired using descriptive statistical methods. For example, as for productive affiliations, the affiliations were ranked according to their decreasing order of productivity. The rankings started with the affiliations with the highest number of diabetes-related publications. We used a publicly available software R for statistical analysis in the paper.

Research hotspots analysis: the recent research hotspots of diabetes in China were acquired based on a keyword co-occurrence matrix with the following steps. (1) Standardization of keywords: there existed nonstandard and inconsistent keyword representations thus it needed to be consistent, e.g., unifying "type 2 diabetes", "diabetes, type 2", "diabetes type 2", "Type 2 diabetes (T2DM)" as "type 2 diabetes"; unifying "type 1 diabetes", "diabetes, type 1", "diabetes type 1", "Type 1 diabetes (T1DM)" as "type 1 diabetes"; unifying "non-insulin-dependent diabetes mellitus", "diabetes, non-insulin-dependent" as "non-insulin-dependent diabetes mellitus"; unifying "Type 1", "TypeI" as "Type 1"; unifying "Type 2", "TypeII" as "Type 2"; unifying "gestational diabetes", "diabetes, pregnancy", "diabetes, gestational" as "gestational diabetes". (2) With the standardization, keywords with high frequency were ranked and sorted. (3) With the top frequent keywords, a co-occurrence matrix was constructed. (4) With the co-occurrence matrix, a keyword correlation matrix was acquired through the calculation using Ochiai correlation coefficient. (5) With the keyword correlation matrix, a keyword dissimilar matrix was generated. (6) Hierarchical clustering and k-means clustering analysis were applied based on the keyword correlation matrix. (7) Multidimensional scaling analysis was implemented based on the keyword dissimilar matrix.

Cooperation network analysis: With the top productive authors and affiliations generated with descriptive statistical method, the cooperation network of authors and affiliations were acquired, respectively. It was required to convert the author and affiliation data into date form of one-to-one cooperation at first, and then the cooperation networks were generated using an easy-to-use package named as *networkD3* in R. It visualized the networks into force-directed graphs using the a function named as *simpleNetwork*.

4   Results and Discussion

As for literature characteristics analysis, the publication date and journal distribution as well as productive affiliations were taken into consideration. Table 1 shows the number and growth rate of diabetes publications by year during 2007–2016, revealing that the total number of publications increased rapidly by year before 2010, but dwindled after 2010. The growth rate of publications on diabetes from 2009 to 2010 reached up to 31.9%, witnessing the great mass upsurge on diabetes research in 2010.

Table 1. The number and growth rate of publications on diabetes by year during 2007–2016

Year	#publications	#cumulative publications	Growth rate (%)
2007	2,202	2,202	–
2008	2,066	4,268	−6.176
2009	2,326	6,594	12.585
2010	3,068	9,662	31.900
2011	2,768	12,430	−9.778
2012	2,337	14,767	−15.571
2013	2,433	17,200	4.108
2014	2,458	19,658	1.028
2015	2,589	22,247	5.330
2016	2,314	24,561	−10.622

The time regression curve of cumulative number of publications could be fitted as $y = -5.075 \times 10^6 + 2.529 \times 10^3 x$ with the goodness-of-fit R^2 equaling to 0.9991. It indicates that the regression curve fitted the development trend of the actual cumulative number of publications well, with which the future research output on diabetes in China could be inferred. For example, the predicted number of publications on diabetes research in 2017 in China is $-5.075 \times 10^6 + 2.529 \times 10^3 \times 2017 - (-5.075 \times 10^6 + 2.529 \times 10^3 \times 2016) = 2529$. Table 2 shows the top 10 most productive journals, from which these 10 journals together accounted for 37.52% of the total publications.

Table 2. Top 10 most productive journals

Journal	#publications	Proportion %	Cumulative proportion %
Chinese Journal of Diabetes	2,431	9.90	9.90
Chinese Journal of Gerontology	1,895	7.71	17.61
Shandong Medical Journal	964	3.92	21.54
Chinese General Practice	885	3.60	25.14
The Journal of Practical Medicine	563	2.29	27.43
Guangdong Medical Journal	520	2.12	29.55
Modern Preventive Medicine	518	2.11	31.66
China Journal of Modern Medicine	495	2.02	33.67
Chongqing Medicine	482	1.96	35.63
Lishizhen Medicine and Material Medical Research	463	1.88	37.52

Table 3 shows the top 10 most productive first author affiliations and total author affiliations, from which *Anhui Provincial Hospital* ranked within top two in both the top 10 most productive first author affiliations and total affiliations, indicating that it contributed much on the diabetes research in China.

Table 3. Top 10 most productive first author affiliations and total affiliations

Rank	First author affiliations	#publications	Rank	Total author affiliations	#publications
1	**Anhui Provincial Hospital**	298	1	Beijing University of Chinese Medicine	641
2	First Affiliated Hospital of Chongqing Medical University	212	2	**Anhui Provincial Hospital**	618
3	General Hospital of PLA	202	3	Guangzhou University of Chinese Medicine	453
4	Shanghai Jiao Tong University Affiliated Sixth People's Hospital	200	4	Shanghai Jiao Tong University Affiliated Sixth People's Hospital	421
5	Nanjing Medical University	187	5	Nanjing Medical University	392
6	Beijing University of Chinese Medicine	177	6	General Hospital of PLA	380
7	First Affiliated Hospital, Nanjing Medical University	160	7	Peking University First Hospital	332
8	Peking University First Hospital	150	8	First Affiliated Hospital of Chongqing Medical University	331
9	Guangzhou University of Chinese Medicine	149	9	Chengdu University of TCM	321
10	Chengdu University of TCM	146	10	First Affiliated Hospital, Nanjing Medical University	276

For the research hotspots analysis, we used author defined keywords. Generally, they can represent the main points of the publications. Table 4 shows 34 keywords with frequency greater than or equaling to 200. The top 3 in order were: "Diabetes" with frequency of 7,510 and frequency of 7.078%, "Type 2 Diabetes" with frequency of 6,978 and frequency of 6.577%, and "Diabetic Nephropathy" with frequency of 2,873 and frequency of 2.708%. Using the keywords, a co-occurrence matrix with 34 rows and 34 columns was generated, where the top 10 keywords are shown as Table 5. The co-occurrence matrix is a symmetric matrix. The data on the main diagonal indicates the frequency of the keywords and the data on the non-main diagonal represents the co-occurrence frequency between two different keywords. For instance, the co-occurrence frequency of "Diabetes" and "Blood Glucose" is 280, indicating that these two keywords appeared together in 280 documents.

Table 4. The ranked keywords with frequency greater than or equaling to 200

Rank	Keyword	Frequency	Frequency %	Rank	Keyword	Frequency	Frequency %
1	Diabetes	7,510	7.078	18	Blood Fat	352	0.332
2	Type 2 Diabetes	6,978	6.577	19	Coronary Heart Disease	321	0.303
3	Diabetic Nephropathy	2,873	2.708	20	Diabetes Rat	315	0.297
4	Insulin Resistance	1,372	1.293	21	Obesity	313	0.295
5	Gestational Diabetes	949	0.894	22	Metformin	283	0.267
6	Blood Glucose	847	0.798	23	C-reactiveprotein	276	0.26
7	Diabetic Retinopathy	752	0.709	24	Fasting Plasma Glucose	266	0.251
8	Diabetic Peripheral Neuropathy	717	0.676	25	Genetic Polymorphism	257	0.242
9	Insulin	625	0.589	26	Acupuncture	252	0.238
10	Oxidative Stress	624	0.588	27	Atherosclerosis	245	0.231
11	Diabetic Foot	595	0.561	28	Streptozotocin	241	0.227
12	Risk Factors	581	0.548	29	Meta Analysis	226	0.213
13	Rat	574	0.541	30	Hypoglycemic	222	0.209
14	Hypertension	522	0.492	31	Metabolic Syndrome	216	0.204
15	Glycosylated Hemoglobin	467	0.44	32	Vascular Endothelial Growth Factor	205	0.193
16	Type 1 Diabetes	407	0.384	33	Diabetic Cardiomyopathy	202	0.19
17	Adiponectin	364	0.343	34	Transforming Growth Factor-β1	201	0.189

After that, we generated a keyword correlation matrix with the basis of the co-occurrence matrix using Ochiai correlation coefficient. The used calculation formula was $O_{ij} = A_{ij}/\sqrt{A_i A_j}$. In the formula, the value range of O_{ij} was [0, 1], representing the probability of the co-occurrence of keyword W_i and W_j. A_{ij} represented the co-occurrence frequency of keyword W_i and W_j. A_i represented the frequency of the keyword W_i and A_j represented the frequency of the keyword W_j. In the correlation matrix, the value represented the distance between two keywords. The larger the

Table 5. The top 10 keywords in the co-occurrence matrix

	Blood Glucose	Diabetes	Diabetic Nephropathy	Diabetic Peripheral Neuropathy	Diabetic Retinopathy	Gestational Diabetes	Insulin	Insulin Resistance	Oxidative Stress	Type2 Diabetes
Blood Glucose	847	280	36	7	4	38	101	36	14	273
Diabetes	280	7,510	109	96	53	6	223	168	143	10
Diabetic Nephropathy	36	109	2,873	3	23	2	10	63	146	235
Diabetic Peripheral Neuropathy	7	96	3	717	2	0	1	2	39	103
Diabetic Retinopathy	4	53	23	2	752	1	1	8	27	92
Gestational Diabetes	38	6	2	0	1	949	43	131	9	4
Insulin	101	223	10	1	1	43	625	33	7	204
Insulin Resistance	36	168	63	2	8	131	33	1,372	40	635
Oxidative Stress	14	143	146	39	27	9	7	40	624	134
Type2 Diabetes	273	10	235	103	92	4	204	635	134	6,978

correlation value was between two keywords, the smaller the distance was between them. Then the keyword dissimilar matrix was acquired through subtracting each value in the correlation matrix from 1.

Therefore, 34 keywords were divided into 7 research hotspot categories through hierarchical clustering, k-means clustering, and multidimensional scaling analysis, respectively. We set the cluster number k as 7 in the experiment from our empirical experience. Figure 2 shows the result of hierarchical clustering using complete-linkage with distance function $D_{HK} = \max(d_{uv})$, $u \in H$ and $v \in K$. d_{uv} represented the distance between word u and v, where u belonged to cluster H and v belonged to cluster K.

Among the generated research hotspot categories using the three methods, three categories are the same as follows: (1) Glycosylated Hemoglobin, and Type 2 Diabetes; (2) Blood Fat, and Blood Glucose; and (3) Diabetic Retinopathy, Vascular Endothelial Growth Factor, Diabetic Nephropathy, and Transforming Growth Factor-β1. Table 6 is a summary of the results of hierarchical clustering, k-means clustering, and multidimensional scaling analysis.

For cooperation network analysis, the number of publications with a specific first author or affiliation was much less than that with cooperation with other authors or affiliations. For example, the number of publications for *Anhui Provincial Hospital* as first author affiliation was 298. However, the number was up to 618 when cooperating with other affiliations, indicating the cooperation among authors or affiliations on diabetes research was much. Therefore, considering all authors in the same publications, we analyzed the cooperation relationships among authors with the number of

Table 6. The summary of the results of hierarchical clustering, k-means clustering, multidimensional scaling analysis

Category	Hierarchical clustering	k-means clustering	Multidimensional scaling analysis
1	**Glycosylated Hemoglobin; Type 2 Diabetes**	**Glycosylated Hemoglobin; Type 2 Diabetes**	**Glycosylated Hemoglobin; Type 2 Diabetes**
2	**Blood Fat; Blood Glucose**	**Blood Fat; Blood Glucose**	**Blood Fat; Blood Glucose**
3	**Diabetic Retinopathy; Vascular Endothelial Growth Factor; Diabetic Nephropathy; Transforming Growth Factor-β1**	**Diabetic Retinopathy; Vascular Endothelial Growth Factor; Diabetic Nephropathy; Transforming Growth Factor-β1**	**Diabetic Retinopathy; Vascular Endothelial Growth Factor; Diabetic Nephropathy; Transforming Growth Factor-β1**
4	Metabolic Syndrome; Obesity; Risk Factors; Coronary Heart Disease; Diabetes; Hypertension; Atherosclerosis; C-reactiveprotein	Metabolic Syndrome; Obesity; Risk Factors; Coronary Heart Disease; Diabetes; Hypertension; Atherosclerosis	Metabolic Syndrome; Obesity; Risk Factors; Coronary Heart Disease; Diabetes; Hypertension; Atherosclerosis; Gestational Diabetes; Type 1 Diabetes; Hypoglycemic; Adiponectin; Insulin Resistance; Insulin
5	Genetic Polymorphism; Meta Analysis; Acupuncture; Diabetic Foot; Fasting Plasma Glucose; Diabetes Rat; Oxidative Stress; Hypoglycemic; Streptozotocin; Type 1 Diabetes;	Genetic Polymorphism; Meta Analysis; Acupuncture; Diabetic Foot; Insulin; Diabetic Peripheral Neuropathy; Metformin; Type 1 Diabetes;	Genetic Polymorphism; Meta Analysis; Acupuncture; Diabetic Foot; Diabetes Rat; Oxidative Stress; Streptozotocin; Diabetic Cardiomyopathy; Fasting Plasma Glucose; C-reactiveprotein; Metformin; Rat
6	Gestational Diabetes; Adiponectin; Insulin Resistance; Insulin; Metformin; Diabetic Cardiomyopathy; Rat	Gestational Diabetes; Adiponectin; Insulin Resistance; C-reactiveprotein	Hypertension
7	Diabetic Peripheral Neuropathy	Hypoglycemic; Fasting Plasma Glucose; Oxidative Stress; Rat; Diabetes Rat; Streptozotocin; Diabetic Cardiomyopathy	Diabetic Peripheral Neuropathy

publications greater than or equaling to 100, 150, and 200, respectively, as well as the affiliations with the number of publications greater than or equaling to 50.

Figure 3 shows the cooperation network of authors with the number of publications >=100 (access via the link[1]). Figure 4 shows the cooperation network of affiliations with the number of publications >=50 (access via the link[2]). In the network, the black

---

[1] http://www.zhukun.org/haoty/resources.asp?id=HIS2017_author_100.

[2] http://www.zhukun.org/haoty/resources.asp?id=HIS2017_affiliation_50.

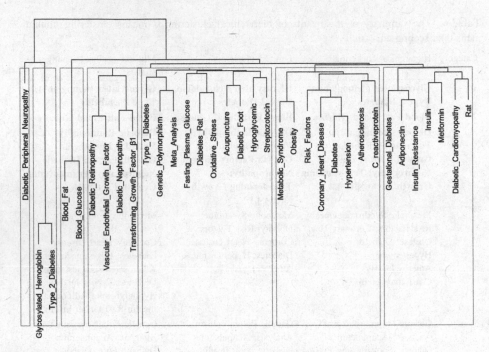

Fig. 2. The visulized result of hierarchical clustering

nodes represent authors or affiliations, and the lines represent the cooperation relationship. The more connected lines surrounding a specific node, the closer cooperation relationship with other authors or affiliations is for the author or affiliation. Moreover, one can dynamically drag and drop to view the cooperation relationship for a specific author or affiliation.

5   Summary

This paper presented a data-driven method based on bibliometrics and knowledge mapping analysis, aiming at discovering the recent research status of diabetes in China during 2007–2016. With the analysis techniques of descriptive statistics, clustering and multidimensional scaling, and network analysis, we acquired literature distribution characteristics, research hotspots, and cooperation relationships among authors and affiliations. The results and findings were presented. Our work can provide clinical researchers and funding agencies with state-of-the-art research status, potentially assisting scientific research topic determination and participating in the development of clinical research strategies.

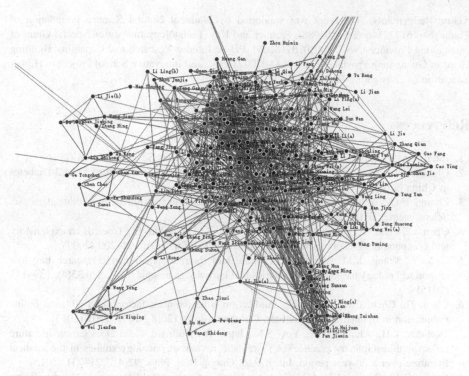

Fig. 3. The cooperation network of authors with the number of publications greater than or equaling to 100

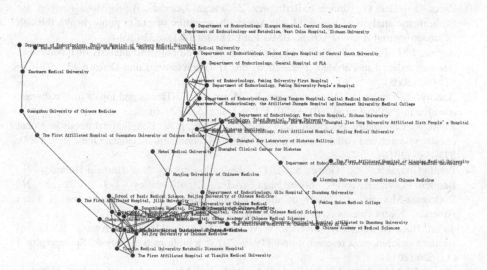

Fig. 4. The cooperation network of affiliations with the number of publications greater than or equaling to 50

Acknowledgements. The work was supported by National Natural Science Foundation of China (No. 61772146 & 61403088), Frontier and Key Technology Innovation Special Grant of Guangdong Province (No. 2014B010118005), Public Interest Research and Capability Building Grant of Guangdong Province (No. 2014A020221039), and Innovative School Project in Higher Education of Guangdong Province (No. YQ2015062).

References

1. International Diabetes Federation (IDF): IDF Diabetes Atlas Seventh Edition (2016)
2. Chinese Diabetes Society: Guidelines for the Prevention and Treatment of Type 2 Diabetes in China (2013). Chin. J. Diabetes Mellitus 6(7) (2014)
3. Zhang, H.Q.: A bibliometric study on medicine chinese traditional in medline database. Scientometrics 31(3), 241–250 (1994)
4. Chen, C., Chen, Y., Horowitz, M., Hou, H., Liu, Z., Pellegrino, D.: Towards an explanatory and computational theory of scientific discovery. J. Infor. 3(3), 191–209 (2009)
5. Guo, Y., Wang, X.M., Wei, H.E.: Chinese and international dynamic research into low carbon technology based on bibliometrics and knowledge mapping. Inf. Sci. 33(4), 139–148 (2015)
6. Chen, H., Chen, C.H., Jhanji, V.: Publication times, impact factors, and advance online publication in ophthalmology journals. Ophthalmology 120(8), 1697–1701 (2013)
7. Holliday, E.B., Ahmed, A.A., Yoo, S.K., Jagsi, R., Hoffman, K.E.: Does cancer literature reflect multidisciplinary practice? A systematic review of oncology studies in the medical literature over a 20-year period. Int. J. Rad. Oncol. Biol. Phys. 92(4), 721–731 (2015)
8. Salisu, S.A., Ojoye, O.T.: Bibliometric analysis of cancer publications in Nigeria during 2008–2012. Int. J. Libr. Inf. Sci. 7(3), 69–76 (2015)
9. Kondilis, B.K., Kiriaze, I.J., Athanasoulia, A.P., Falagas, M.E.: Mapping health literacy research in the European Union: a bibliometric analysis. PLoS ONE 3(6), e2519 (2008)
10. Zacca-González, G., Chinchilla-Rodríguez, Z., Vargas-Quesada, B., de Moya-Anegón, F.: Bibliometric analysis of regional Latin America's scientific output in public health through SCImago journal & country rank. BMC Publ. Health 14(1), 632 (2014)
11. Ramos, J.M., Padilla, S., Masia, M., Gutierrez, F.: A bibliometric analysis of tuberculosis research indexed in PubMed, 1997–2006. Int. J. Tuberculosis Lung Disease 12, 121461–121468 (2008)
12. Boudry, C., Denion, E., Mortemousque, B., Mouriaux, F.: Trends and topics in eye disease research in PubMed from 2010 to 2014. PeerJ 4, e1557 (2016)
13. Khan, A., Choudhury, N., Uddin, S., Hossain, L., Baur, L.A.: Longitudinal trends in global obesity research and collaboration: a review using bibliometric metadata. Obes. Rev. 17(4), 377–385 (2016)
14. Perilla-González, Y., Gómez-Suta, D., Delgado-Osorio, N., Hurtado-Hurtado, N., Baquero-Rodriguez, J.D., Lopez-Isaza, A.F., Lagos-Grisales, G.J., Villegas, N., Rodriguez-Morales, A.: Study of the scientific production on leishmaniasis in Latin America. Recent Patents Anti Infective Drug Disc. 9(3), 216–222 (2014)
15. Sa'ed, H.Z., Al-Jabi, S.W., Sweileh, W.M., Al-Khalil, S., Alqub, M., Awang, R.: Global methaemoglobinaemia research output (1940–2013): a bibliometric analysis. Springerplus 4(1), 626 (2015)
16. Escobedo, A.A., Arencibia, R., Vega, R.L., Rodríguez-Morales, A.J., Almirall, P., Alfonso, M.: A bibliometric study of international scientific productivity in giardiasis covering the period 1971–2010. J. Infection Developing Countries 9(1), 076–086 (2015)

17. Man, H., Xin, S., Bi, W., Lv, C., Mauro, T.M., Elias, P.M., Man, M.Q.: Comparison of publication trends in dermatology among Japan, South Korea and Mainland China. BMC Dermatol. **14**(1), 1 (2014)
18. Gao, Y., Qu, B., Shen, Y., Su, X.J., Dong, X.Y., Chen, X.M., Pi, H.Y.: Bibliometric profile of neurogenic bladder in the literature: a 20-year bibliometric analysis. Neural Regener. Res. **10**(5), 797 (2015)
19. Cheng, T., Zhang, G.: Worldwide research productivity in the field of rheumatology from 1996 to 2010: a bibliometric analysis. Rheumatology **52**(9), 1630–1634 (2013). ket008
20. Sharma, B., Boet, S., Grantcharov, T., Shin, E., Barrowman, N.J., Bould, M.D.: The h-index outperforms other bibliometrics in the assessment of research performance in general surgery: a province-wide study. Surgery **153**(4), 493–501 (2013)
21. Harande, Y.I.: Exploring the literature of diabetes in Nigeria: a bibliometrics study. Afr. J. Diabetes Med. **19**(2), 1–4 (2011)
22. Harande, Y.I., Alhaji, I.U.: Basic literature of diabetes: a bibliometrics analysis of three countries in different world regions. J. Libr. Inf. Sci. **2**(1), 49–56 (2014)
23. Nasli-Esfahani, E., Farzadfar, F., Kouhnavard, M., Ghodssi-Ghassemabadi, R., Khajavi, A., Peimani, M., Sanjari, M.: Iran diabetes research roadmap (IDRR) study: a preliminary study on diabetes research in the world and Iran. J. Diabetes Metabolic Disorders **16**(1), 9 (2017)
24. Geaney, F., Scutaru, C., Kelly, C., Glynn, R.W., Perry, I.J.: Type 2 diabetes research yield, 1951–2012: bibliometrics analysis and density-equalizing mapping. PLoS ONE **10**(7), e0133009 (2015)
25. Zhang, Y., Shen, X., Chen, D.: Bibliometrics analysis of the relationship research of antipsychotics and type 2 diabetes. Chin. J. Drug Dependence **1**, 19 (2011)

Generation of Semantic Patient Data for Depression

Yanan Du[1(✉)], Shaofu Lin[1], and Zhisheng Huang[2]

[1] School of Software Engineering, Beijing University of Technology, Beijing, China
duyanan56@emails.bjut.edu.cn, linshaofu@bjut.edu.cn
[2] Department of Computer Science, VU University Amsterdam, Amsterdam, The Netherlands
huang@cs.vu.nl

Abstract. In the medicine practice, due to the privacy and safety of electronic medical record (EMR), the sharing, research and application of EMR have been hindered to a certain extent. Thus, it becomes increasingly important to study semantic electronic medical data integration, so as to meet the needs of doctors and researchers and help them quickly access high-quality information. This paper focuses on the realization of semantic EMRs. It shows how to uses APDG (Advanced Patient Data Generator) to create a set of virtual patient data for depression. Furthermore, it explains how to develop clinical and semantic description rules to construct semantic EMRs for depression and discusses how those generated virtual patient data can be used in the system of Smart Ward for the test and demonstration, without violating the legal issues (e.g., privacy and security) of patient data.

Keywords: Semantic technology · Electronic medical record · Data integration · Depression

1 Introduction

Depression is a common but serious mood disorder with high recurrence and high suicide rate [1]. According to the World Health Organization (WHO), depression is the world's fourth largest disease. It is expected that by 2020, depression will become the second largest disease after cardiovascular disease [2]. In China, the incidence of depression is about 6%, while the number of diagnosis of depression is nearly 30 million. Because mental illness involves lots of privacy data, further research on depression is quite limited. In the future treatment of depression, it is important for doctors and researchers to improve the cognition of depression.

The EMR is a complete and detailed clinical information resource which generated in the course of medical treatment. As early as 1997, an American Richard S. Dick made a clear statement: EMR is not just about using the computer to transplant the paper records into electronic carriers. Moreover, it changes the text and chart information into the formatted data, which can not only be recognized and understood by computer but also be entered, stored, processed, and inquired [3]. According to the above description, there are two main types of EMR, in which one is based on the structure and the other is based on the semantic technology.

S. Siuly et al. (Eds.): HIS 2017, LNCS 10594, pp. 102–112, 2017.
https://doi.org/10.1007/978-3-319-69182-4_11

Although structured EMR provides a syntactic norm, it does not specify the structure and semantics of clinical documents. What is more, it is difficult to carry out the precise query of the content and realize the intelligent processing (e.g., semantic reasoning). Besides, it cannot guarantee the interoperability between the systems, which will lead to low utilization.

As a comprehensive knowledge modeling technology, semantic technology uses semantic-based expression language with international standards, such as RDF data and OWL ontology language [4]. At present, semantic technology has been widely used in many fields. It offers important technical support for intelligent analysis and clinical decision of information system. The European Union proposed in the *Semantic Interoperability for Better Health and Safer Healthcare* that, semantic interoperability is essential for improving the quality as well as the safety of care, public health, and clinical research [5]. Therefore, how to use information technology to obtain and improve the value of EMR is one of the crucial issues for people's health and medical development.

The Advanced Patient Data Generator (APDG) [6] is a knowledge-based approach of synthesizing large scale patient data. The basic rationale for this synthesis is to make the generated patient data look like realistic as possible as we could, by using various domain knowledge to control the patient data generation. APDG provides a tool to create semantic patient data, more exactly RDF Ntriple data, for both realistic and virtual patents. In this paper, we will show how to use the APDG tool to generate a set of semantic patient data for virtual patients of depression, and how to develop clinical and semantic description rules to construct those semantic EMRs for depression. Furthermore, we will discuss how those generated virtual patient data for depression can be used in the system of Smart Ward of Depression for the purpose of system tests and demonstration, without violating the legal issues (e.g., privacy and security) of patient data.

The rest of this paper is organized as follows. Section 2 gives an overview of related works. Section 3 elaborates knowledge Integration and rule expression of semantic EMR. Section 4 illustrates the data integration of EMR for depression. Section 5 proposes the application of semantic EMR. The last section includes conclusions and future work.

2   Related Work

In recent years, with the integration of information technology and medical industry, the intelligent analysis and application of EMR have become increasingly significant. Based on the development of medical information integration technology, many researchers have proposed to enhance EMR's application performance with the advanced information technologies.

Based on clinical workflow, Alessio Bottrighi et al. presented evaluation and development of clinical guidelines and medical knowledge. By carrying out the configuration of clinical information system, they successfully evaluated the physician's behavior and provided alarm information to clinicians [7]. Dimitrios Alexandrou et al. developed the SEMPATH system prototype which contained the required knowledge ontology framework. The clinical path adaptive capability could be achieved through workflow management and rule libraries [8–10]. BioDASH refers to a Semantic Web prototype of a Drug Development Dashboard that associates disease, compounds, molecular biology, and pathway knowledge for a team of users. Additionally, the project used rule-based processing technology and RDF reasoning engine to implement rule-based filtering and integration for clinical data [11].

In China, the development of EMR has just begun. Due to the inconsistencies of the standard system as well as the constraints of policies and laws, it is difficult to implement the integration and sharing of data. As a result, EMR cannot provide a wider range of medical services, medical researches, and other functions [12].

However, there is still a large room for growth in EMR. Firstly, EMR can be made to improve the quality of medical services and offer decision support by data collection, analysis, and utilization. Secondly, EMR can provide hospital leaders or clinicians with useful information and decision-making through data modeling, prediction, and processing [13].

3 Knowledge Integration and Rule Expression of Semantic EMR

3.1 Advanced Patient Data Generator

In this study, APDG is used to synthesize large-scale patient data. APDG can support a comprehensive domain knowledge description and variable control, provide a powerful and convenient function to generate various patient data, and meet different requirements. In addition, the Patient Data Definition Language (PDDL) defined by APDG is designed based on the XML format. It controls the data generation process by defining the patient's general format data, and the generated data can be flexibly converted to other data formats [6]. Figure 1 illustrates the architecture of APDG.

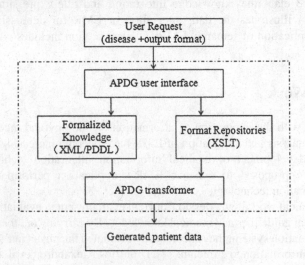

Fig. 1. The architecture of APDG

3.2 Knowledge and Rule

To make the generated patient data as realistic as possible, we controlled the data generation process by using domain knowledge and general knowledge. Collected knowledge is formalized in the PDDL for the patient data generation. More specifically, domain knowledge is related to a particular disease (depression), which includes gender distribution, the average duration, clinical symptoms, incentives, and suicide rate. General knowledge is independent of domain knowledge, which involves the number of patient's medical record, native place, address, and occupation. Domain knowledge is mainly collected from the following resources.

Biomedical publications. Biomedical publications and medical books provide rich information about diseases and patients. The description of depression in the *Guidelines for the Prevention and Treatment of Depression* can be listed as follows [14]. Table 1 shows the proportions of somatopathy symptoms in depression patients.

Table 1. Somatic disease and proportion

Symptom	Proportion
Sleep disorder	98%
Fatigue	83%
Appetite disorder	71%
Constipation	67%
Weight loss	63%
Headache	42%
Gastrointestinal symptoms	36%

The average age of depression is 20 to 30 years old, the average duration is 16 weeks, and the recurrence rate is about 35%. Among depression patients, 75%–80% had the idea of suicide, and about 20% choose to commit suicide.

Network resources. Network resources such as Wikipedia and Medical Websites usually provide information about the distribution of diseases and its dependence on other variables (e.g. gender, age, etc.).

The gender distribution of depression is about 1:2 (male to female). The number of women who had a positive family history was twice that of men. A study by the World Federation of Mental Health (WFMH) shows that 69% of patients who were diagnosed with depression had unexplained somatic symptoms during the treatment process.

Professional EHR reference. Experts at Beijing Anding Hospital provided us with information about depression, EMR and other professional information.

4   Data Integration of Semantic EMR

4.1   XML Definition

In this paper, the international standardized semantic description language (RDF) has been used to integrate semantic data. The RDF format, which can be applied independently, directly, and legibly, is used to describe information flexibly with the minimal constraints.

Generally, the EMR can be divided into two sections. To be specific, one is the external feature, which includes the patient's basic information (name, sex, address etc.). The other is internal feature, which describes the course of disease, including complaints, history of past illness, psychological examination and so on [15].

Based on the APDG, we have constructed the model and standardized XML Schema document of EMR, which can be used to restrict it on structure and semantics. Finally, a set of virtual patient data was created for depression. To ensure the rationality and availability of data, we focused on the association between feature information and resources contained in EMR. For completing data integration and storage, we accessed to relevant domain knowledge and experts' advice from Beijing Anding Hospital, and verified it repeatedly.

```xml
<Slot value="incentives">
<DataRange>
<Distributions type="enumeration" variable="$incentives">
  <Distribution item="No obvious incentive" pfrom="0"
pto="40"/>
  <Distribution item="Serious illness of family members"
pfrom="40" pto="45"/>
  <Distribution item="Death of family members" pfrom="45"
pto="50"/>
  <Distribution item="work pressure" pfrom="50" pto="58"/>
  <Distribution item="unemployment" pfrom="58" pto="66"/>
  <Distribution item="Relationship breakup" pfrom="66"
pto="70">
  <Distribution item="divorce" pfrom="70" pto="74"
condition="$birthyear =< 1986 AND $birthyear => 1956"/>
  <Distribution item="marital discord" pfrom="74" pto="78"
condition="$birthyear =< 1986 AND $birthyear => 1956"/>
  <Distribution item="widowed" pfrom="78" pto="85"
condition="$birthyear =< 1986 AND $birthyear => 1956"/>
  <Distribution item="serious physical illness" pfrom="85"
pto="92" condition="$birthyear =< 1996 AND $birthyear => 1956"/>
  <Distribution item="accident" pfrom="92" pto="100"/>
</Distributions>
</DataRange>
</Slot>
```

In this study, we can specify the integrated number of EMRs. Furthermore, each EMR has its own patient ID, the aim of which is to ensure that the generated data can be uniquely identified. The data format supports several formats of RDF data, which include the Ntriple data format and RDF/XML data format. Here are the examples of how we generated data from XML constraints:

Incentive. The following proportional control is based on common incentives of depression.

Gender. According to domain knowledge, we know that the ratio of the gender distribution of depression patients is 2:1 (female to male). Thus, we set the gender to 'female' with 66% and 'male' with 34%. The knowledge of the gender distribution of depression can be specified as a rule of PDDL as follows:

```
<Slot value="Gender">
<DataRange>
<enumeration value="male"/>
<enumeration value="female"/>
  <Distributions type="enumeration" variable="$gender">
    <Distribution item="male" pfrom="66" pto="100"/>
    <Distribution item="female" pfrom="0" pto="66"/>
  </Distributions>
</DataRange>
</Slot>
```

4.2 Semantic Annotation

Metadata is descriptive information about data and information resources [16]. Medical metadata is able to describe the collection of data items needed by specific objects in the field of medicine and health, as well as the semantic definitions of each data item. Also, it can be applied to data collection, reuse, distribution, and query in the medical and health field. Medical metadata for EMR includes Unified Medical Language System (UMLS), Systematized Nomenclature of Medicine (SNOMED), etc. The Systematized Nomenclature of Medicine-Clinical Term (SNOMED CT) relates to a core generic term set in the field of e-health with a unique meaning. Based on the defined hierarchy, it contains 19 levels of systems and more than 311,000 independent concepts. There are approximately 1,360,000 semantic associations [17].

After completing the knowledge representation and XML constraints, we used SNOMED[1] to manually annotate the medical metadata contained in the document. Semantic annotation means annotating of natural language texts into their corresponding medical ontologies so that they can interoperate with other semantic data. The key to realizing semantic interoperability is to solve the consistency of understanding the same concept between systems. Applying SNOMED CT to annotate EMR data is to ensure the consistency of the meanings of clinical medical terms and to lay the foundation for future research.

---

[1] http://www.snomebrowser.com/.

We defined concept mapping rules in PDDL to make the semantic annotations on the slots/properties of patient data for data integration. For example, the following rule is used to make the semantic annotation on the slots gender, male, and female with their corresponding concept IDs in medical ontology SNOMED CT:

```
<Slot value="Gender">
<ConceptMapping ontology="snomed" conceptid="263495000"/>
<DataRange>
<enumeration value="male"/>
<ConceptMapping ontology="snomed" conceptid="703117000"/>
<enumeration value="female"/>
<ConceptMapping ontology="snomed" conceptid="703118005"/>
  <Distributions type="enumeration" variable="$gender">
    ......
  </Distributions>
</DataRange>
</Slot>
```

5   Experiments and Applications

5.1   Data Storage

As we have discussed above, APDG is used to generate data for the semantic EMRs in RDF NTriple format. In this case, we have generated 1,000 patient data with the first diagnostic of depression, which covers the primary characteristics of patients who are diagnosed with depression for the first time. Below is part of the NTriple files of the generated semantic EMR.

```
<http://wasp.cs.vu.nl/apdg#> <http://www.w3.org/2000/01/rdf-
schema#label> "Patient ID".
<http://wasp.cs.vu.nl/apdg#> <http://wasp.cs.vu.nl/apdg#value>
"MDD_DYN20161000000".
<http://wasp.cs.vu.nl/apdg#> <http://www.w3.org/2000/01/rdf-
schema#label> "Gender".
<http://wasp.cs.vu.nl/apdg#> <http://wasp.cs.vu.nl/apdg#Concept>
<http://www.ihtsdo.org/SCT_263495000>
<http://wasp.cs.vu.nl/apdg#> <http://wasp.cs.vu.nl/apdg#value>
"female".
<http://wasp.cs.vu.nl/apdg#> <http://www.w3.org/2000/01/rdf-
schema#label> "main Complain".
<http://wasp.cs.vu.nl/apdg#> <http://wasp.cs.vu.nl/apdg#value>
"Accompanied by Headache and long-term depression for two years".
```

According to the statistics, we integrated 1000 EMR data which contains 165,000 triples. The number of semantic annotation is 28,000. Due to the particularity of depression, several descriptions of EMR (e.g., psychological examination) cannot completely correspond to the concept in SNOMED. Those generated 1,000 EMR data, which can be loaded into any triple store for semantic query, can be further used for an application system of semantic technology. We have loaded the semantic patient data in GraphDB[2] and the LarKC platform, a semantic platform for scalable semantic data processing [18]. GraphDB is a database which resides inside SQL Server together with a set of.Net 4.5 assemblies partitioned into a client and an admin API (Application Programming Interface). Figure 2 shows a screen shot of the generated EMRs in the interface of GraphDB, a graph database system for the storage and the semantic querying over the semantic EMR data. GraphDB is a powerful system for graph-based semantic queries. Compared with relational databases, graph databases directly store the relationships between records, and they can scale more naturally to large data sets as they do not typically need costly join operations.

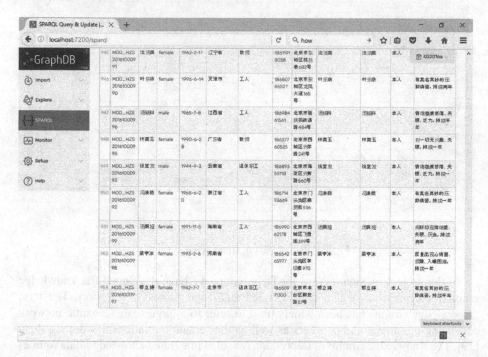

Fig. 2. Patient data in GraphDB

5.2 Applications

The resulting semantic EMRs have been applied to the project of Smart Ward, funded by National Natural Science Foundation of China for a major international cooperation

---

[2] http://graphdb.ontotext.com/graphdb/.

project between Beijing University of Technology and VU University Amsterdam. The Smart Ward project aims to develop a knowledge-based platform for monitoring and analyzing patients' status and providing clinicians or medical researchers with knowledge integration and support of clinical decision. Meanwhile, it will be applied and evaluated in Beijing Anding Hospital, one of the biggest psychiatric hospitals in China. Therefore, we develop the interface system in Chinese. Figure 3 shows a screen shot of the generated EMRs in the interface of the Smart Ward System. The results show that the generated patient data are useful for the tests in the system.

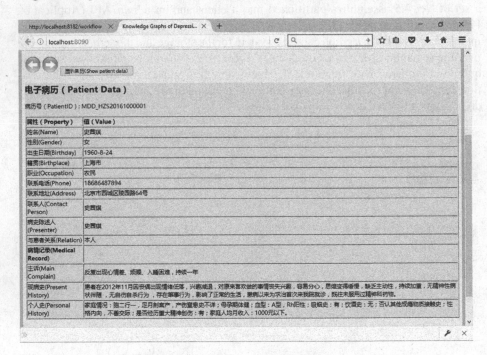

Fig. 3. Patient data in smart ward system

In the project of Smart Ward for Depression, we have developed the knowledge graphs of depression, which is also called as "DepressionKG" for short. The term "Knowledge Graph" has been widely used to refer to a large scale semantic network consisting of entities and concepts as well as the semantic relationships among them [19]. The Knowledge Graphs of Depression is a set of integrated knowledge/data sources concerning depression. It provides the data infrastructure which can be used to explore the relationship among various knowledge/data sources of depression and support for clinical/medical decision support systems. DepressionKG is represented with the format RDF/NTriple. The generated EMRs of depression have been integrated and included in the current version of Knowledge Graphs of Depression [20].

6   Conclusion and Future Work

EMRs are not only the important medical information resources but also the basis of clinical medical information. EMRs contain a large amount of information, such as medical information, everyday language, and other descriptive natural language.

This paper explores how to achieve the data integration of patients using the semantic technology, and how to utilize APDG to generate semantic patient data for depression patients. Those generated patient data is conducive to medical research of researchers as well as sharing and interoperability of EMRs.

For the current study, the existing defined PDDL rules for APDG are still not yet fine-grained to make comprehensive semantic annotations of generated patient data for depression. We will continue to work out more detailed and more fine-grained rules for semantic annotation, so that the generated virtual patient data would look like realistic ones. We will make the evaluation of the generated patient data with professionals in medical domain. We leave this work as one of the future work. Furthermore, we will generate more virtual patient data, not only for those with the first diagnoses, but also for those in-patients with more details of medication and other information in a ward.

References

1. Sullivan, P.F., Neale, M.C., Kendler, K.S.: Genetic epidemiology of major depression: review and meta-analysis. Am. J. Psychiatry **157**(10), 1552–1562 (2000)
2. Reddy, M.S.: Depression: the disorder and the burden. Indian J. Psychol. Med. **32**(1), 1 (2010)
3. Detmer, D.E., Steen, E.B., Dick, R.S. (eds.): The Computer-Based Patient Record: An Essential Technology for Health Care. National Academies Press, Washington (1997)
4. Hitzler, P., Krotzsch, M., Rudolph, S.: Foundations of semantic web technologies. CRC Press, Boca Raton (2009)
5. European Commission. Semantic interoperability for better health and safer healthcare. Deployment and research roadmap for Europe. ISBN-13: 978-92- 79-11139-6; 2009
6. Huang, Z., van Harmelen, F., ten Teije, A., et al.: Knowledge-based patient data generation. In: Riaño, D., Lenz, R., Miksch, S., Peleg, M., Reichert, M., ten Teije, A. (eds.) KR4HC/ProHealth 2013. LNCS, vol. 8268, pp. 83–96. Springer, Cham (2013). doi: 10.1007/978-3-319-03916-9_7
7. Bottrighi, A., Chesani, F., Mello, P., Molino, G., Montali, M., Montani, S., Storari, S., Terenziani, P., Torchio, M.: A hybrid approach to clinical guideline and to basic medical knowledge conformance. Proc. Artif. Intell. Med. **5651**, 91–95 (2009)
8. Alexandrou, D., Xenikoudakis, F., Mentzas, G.: Adaptive clinical pathway with semantic web rules. In: Proceedings of the First International Conference on Health Informatics (2008)
9. Alexandrou, D., Skitsas, I., Mentzas, G.: A holistic environment for the design and execution of self_adaptive clinical pathways. In: Proceeding of the 9th International Conference on Information Technology and Applications in Biomedicine (2009)
10. Alexandrou, D., Xenikoudakis, F., Mentzas, G.: SEMPATH: semantic adaptive and personalized clinical pathways. In: International Conference on eHealth, Telemedicine and Social Medicine (2009)
11. Neumann, E., Quan, D.: BioDASH: a semantic web dashboard for drug development. Pac. Symp. Biocomput. **11**, 176–187 (2006)

12. PengLi, X.: Analysis on the development of electronic medical records in China. Chinese Med. Rec. **5**, 46–47 (2013). (In Chinese)

13. Ma, X., Yang, G., Jingjie, Yu.: Analysis on the development and application of domestic electronic medical records. Comput. Appl. Softw. **32**(1), 10–12 (2015). (In Chinese)

14. Li, L., Ma, X.: Guidelines for the prevention and treatment of Depression. Chinese Medical Electronic Audio and Video Publishing House, pp. 10–36 (2015)

15. Hayrinen, K., Saranto, K., Nykanen, P.: Definition, structure, content, use and impacts of electronic health records: a review of the research literature. Int. J. Med. Inform. **77**, 291–304 (2008)

16. Al-Khalifa, H.S., Davis, H.C.: The evolution of metadata from standards to semantics in E-learning applications. In: Proceedings of the Seventeenth Conference on Hypertext and Hypermedia, pp. 69–72. ACM (2006)

17. Elkin, P.L., Brown, S.H., Husser, C.S., et al.: Evaluation of the content coverage of SNOMED CT: ability of SNOMED clinical terms to represent clinical problem lists. In: Mayo Clinic Proceedings. Elsevier, vol. 81(6), pp. 741–748 (2006)

18. Cheptsov, A., Assel, M., Gallizo, G., et al.: Large knowledge collider. A service-oriented platform for large-scale semantic reasoning. In: Proceedings of the International Conference on Web Intelligence, Mining and Semantics (WIMS 2011), ACM International Conference Proceedings Series, Sogndal, Norway (2011)

19. Singhal, A.: Introducing the Knowledge Graph: Things, Not Strings. Official Google Blog (2012)

20. Huang, Z., Yang, J., van Harmelen, F., Hu, Q.: Constructing disease-centric knowledge graphs: a case study for depression (short version). In: Proceedings of the 2017 International Conference on Artificial Intelligence in Medicine (2017)

Analyses of the Dual Immune Roles Cytokines Play in Ischemic Stroke

Yingying Wang[1,2], Jianfeng Liu[3], Haibo Yu[4], and Yunpeng Cai[1,2(✉)]

[1] Research Center for Biomedical Information Technology, Shenzhen Institutes of Advanced Technology, Chinese Academy of Sciences, Shenzhen, China
yp.cai@siat.ac.cn
[2] Shenzhen Engineering Laboratory of Health Big Data Analyses Technology, Shenzhen, China
[3] Department of Neurology, The First Affiliated Hospital of Harbin Medical University, Harbin, China
[4] Shenzhen Traditional Chinese Medicine Hospital, Shenzhen, China

Abstract. Stroke is one of the leading causes of morbidity and permanent disability worldwide. There is a need for an efficacious alternative therapy administered beyond the limitation of time window based on the biological characteristics of stroke, currently. The immunomodulatory therapy could extend the time window while not increase the risk of hemorrhage which made it become candidate treatments. In this paper, we integrated several gene expression profiles generated from the peripheral blood of ischemic stroke patients and health people. Differential expressed cytokines were first selected as candidate cytokines. Enrichment analyses were then performed to filter the candidate cytokines as biomarkers (E-CKs) by checking the relationships between them and the stroke related functional terms. More cytokines were found as biomarkers in the subacute stage of ischemic stroke compared with acute and chronic stages which could be explained by the great changes in microenvironment in this necrosis stage. Analyses based on microRNomics level showed that more E-CKs one miRNA regulated, the more important role it played in stroke related processes. Similarly, analyses on proteomics level showed that E-CKs with top degrees in the protein-protein interaction network were proved to be closely related to stroke. Most E-CKs participate in both the stroke processing and rehabilitation, thus, the dual immune characters made them become valuable potential targets of immunomodulatory therapies.

Keywords: Cytokine · Ischemic stroke · Dual immune roles

1   Introduction

Stroke is one of the leading causes of morbidity and permanent disability worldwide. Over 70% of all cases are ischemic stroke (IS). As the most widely accepted and used treatment of IS in clinic, the main drawbacks of recombinant tissue plasminogen

---

Y. Wang and J. Liu contributed equally to this paper.

© Springer International Publishing AG 2017
S. Siuly et al. (Eds.): HIS 2017, LNCS 10594, pp. 113–120, 2017.
https://doi.org/10.1007/978-3-319-69182-4_12

activator (rt-PA) are the narrow therapeutic time window (4.5 h), and the consequent increased risk of intracranial hemorrhage which made only a few stroke patients benefit from this therapy [1–3]. Therefore, there is a need for an efficacious alternative therapy administered beyond the limitation of time window based on the biological character- istics of stroke [4, 5]. Currently, many researches indicated that the complication of IS is partly caused by the mutual interplay between central nervous system (CNS) and immune system, especially innate immune response, which plays a dual role by bring different effects on the outcome [6]. The immunomodulatory therapy could extend the time window since inflammatory responses require hours to days to fulfill compared with the immediately reacts after ischemic onset. Meanwhile, the treatment based on immunomodulatory will not increase the risk of hemorrhage. However, the longer time window and the dual character of immune system make the filtrations of biomarkers complicated. The key to this problem is the suitable type of biomarkers.

As the one type of the most investigated inflammatory mediators, cytokines were produced by the infiltrating and active innate immune cells. These cytokines often exhibit dual characters reflected by exacerbating or alleviating inflammatory damages to the ischemic tissue. Thus, cytokines could be chosen as biomarkers which are the basis and potential targets of immunomodulatory therapies. Former researches have validated cytokines such as IL-1 [7, 8], IL-6 [9, 10], and TNF- α [11, 12] play important roles in IS by affecting the infarct volume and tissue damage. However, systematic analyses of cytokines in IS based on their dual immune roles at different time points were still lacking.

Integrative analyses based on multiple 'omics were widely accepted in bioinfor- matics. Following the central dogma, it is of great importance to combine datasets covering genomics, transcriptomics, and proteomics together in order to perform systematic analyses on complex diseases such as stroke. Besides, miRNAs were found to be involved in a number of diseases including stroke by binding to their targets in many researches [13–17]. Thus, the import of microRNomics is necessary. In this paper, we integrated several microarray datasets with samples from IS patients' and health controls' blood at different time points. Differential expressed cytokines between different time points were first selected as candidate cytokines. Enrichment analyses were then performed to filter the candidate cytokines by checking their enrichments in the related functional terms and results showed that these cytokines were tended to involve more in sub-acute stage. Analyses based on microRNomics indicated us that the more E-CKs one miRNA regulated, the more likely it is involved in stroke related processes. The analyses from proteomics showed that the cytokines interact with more other cytokines are more likely to play a key role in stroke. Most cytokines had dual immune character, thus, the dual role made them become valuable potential targets of immunomodulatory therapies.

2   Materials and Methods

2.1   Microarray Datasets and Normalization

We downloaded three microarray datasets from NCBI GEO [18] (See Table 1). The samples of the three datasets were blood from stroke patients at different time points.

Table 1.   Microarray datasets information.

GEO series ID	GEO platform ID	Number of probes
GSE58294	GPL570	54676
GSE37587	GPL6883	24527
GSE22255	GPL570	54676
GSE58294	GPL570	54676
GSE37587	GPL6883	24527

Dataset GSE58294 [19] contained 69 stroke blood samples analyzed at 3 time points: less than 3 h (without treatment), 5 h (after treatment), and 24 h (after treatment) following the event. 23 samples were collected at each time points and divided into 2 sub-datasets and the 23 samples in the control group were also considered as 1 sub-dataset. Dataset GSE37587 [20] contained 68 stroke blood samples analyzed at 2 time points: 24 h and 24–48 h. 34 samples were collected at each time points and divided into 2 sub-datasets. Dataset GSE22255 [21] contained 20 stroke blood samples after 6 months since the patients got the first stroke and 20 controls. Then GSE22255 was considered to be divided into 2 sub-datasets.

All the probes were mapped to gene symbols and mean values were calculated as the expression values if multiple probes were mapped to a same gene. Common genes among the gene sets were chosen to perform the analyses. Then min-max normalization was used for each sub-dataset. For each gene (g_i) in each sub-dataset, the normalized value of the gene in each sample is calculated as follows:

$$\text{Normalized}(g_i) = \frac{g_i - G_{min}}{G_{max} - G_{min}}$$

where G_{min} and G_{max} are the minimum and maximum values for the gene in all the samples, correspondingly.

Then we combined 2 sub-datasets got samples at 24 h of stroke in GSE58294 and GSE37587 into one dataset. The 2 control samples groups in GSE58294 and GSE22255 were also combined into one dataset. Taken together, we got 5 sub-datasets marked as "stroke-5 h (23 samples), stroke-24 h (57 samples), stroke-48 h (34 samples), stroke-6mon (20 samples), healthy (43 samples)", correspondingly. These datasets could be further grouped to the following stages according to pathological stages [22]: (1) acute stage: 5 h after the ischemic onset; (2) sub-acute/necrosis stage: 24 and 48 h after the ischemic onset; and (3) convalescent/chronic stage: 6 months after the ischemic onset.

2.2 Functional Terms

Cytokine-related Functional Terms. The functional datasets were downloaded from GSEA MSigDB database V5.0 [23]. All the datasets containing 'cytokine' as one key word were selected as the 'cytokine-related functional terms' in this study.

Human Protein-Protein Interaction Network. The human protein-protein interaction network composed of 9674 nodes and 39240 edges was downloaded from HPRD [24].

miRNA-Gene Relationships. The 322391 validated miRNA-gene targeting relationships between 2650 miRNAs and 14852 genes were downloaded from miRTarBase v6.1 [25].

2.3 Differential Expression Analyses

Student t-test was used to perform the differential expression analyses for the common genes in the data sets. The genes differentially expressed in the following pairs were considered as process-related DEGs (Differential Expressed Genes) since they were involved in the developments of IS: stroke-5 h vs. stroke-24 h, stroke-24 h vs. stroke-48 h, stroke-48 h vs. stroke-6mon, and stroke-6mon vs. healthy. Compared with this, the genes differentially expressed in the following pairs were considered as recovery-related DEGs since they reflect the gene expression changes between stroke key time points and healthy conditions: stroke-5 h vs. healthy, stroke-24 h vs. healthy, stroke-48 h vs. healthy, and stroke-6mon vs. healthy.

2.4 Enrichment Analyses

Enrichment analyses using one-side Fisher's exact test were performed for all the DEGs on all the cytokine-related functional terms. Each functional term that was enriched by at least one DEG set was considered as an enriched functional term under the corresponding stages. The DEGs in the enriched functional term were marked as E-CK in this study.

3 Results and Discussion

3.1 Differential Expressed Cytokine Genes

There were 14462 common genes among the datasets we used in this study. With threshold 0.05, the numbers of E-CKs of different levels were listed in Table 2. As shown in former studies, the expression of genes changed rapidly after the ischemic onset. In this study, we found that the 7.49%, 5.57% of the whole DEGs with dual immune roles were E-CKs, respectively. This indicated us that the cytokines were interesting biomarkers with both process-related and recovery-related characteristics. It was interesting that no cytokine was found to be differentially expressed between chronic and healthy (See Table 2 for details), which may be explained by the phenomenon that the number of inflammatory related processes in the chronic stage (normally 6 months after the ischemic onset) were smaller compared with the other two stages because most necrotic tissue has been removed.

Table 2. Numbers of DEGs on different levels.

	Stage1 vs. Stage2	Number of E-CKs
Process related	Acute vs. Sub-acute	171
	Sub-acute vs. Chronic	145
Recovery related	Acute vs. healthy	137
	Sub-acute vs. healthy	227
	Chronic vs. healthy	0

As shown in Table 2, the cytokines were tended to involve more in sub-acute stage. This could be explained by the great changes in the microenvironment in this necrosis stage as follows: a large number of nerve cells were lost, glial cells were broken, neutrophils, lymphocytes and macrophages were infiltrated, and the brain tissue became edematous, etc. Thus, cytokines may play important roles in these procedures indicating that more attention should be paid on this stage which may help find new treatment markers in clinic.

3.2   miRNAs as Regulators of E-CKs

Each miRNA got a score by counting the number of E-CKs as its target gene. 181 miRNAs were found to regulate at least one E-CK. The relationships between IS and miRNAs with over 10 E-CKs as target genes were checked using bibliography retrieval. Only hsa-miR-148b-3p was not proved by any research as a biomarker for stroke. The other 7 miRNAs were all be validated to be involved in stroke by researches as follows: hsa-miR-335-5p was shown to bring about a beneficial outcome in IS [26]. hsa-miR-26b-5p was involved in inflammation in atrial fibrillation, which is an important risk factor for stroke [27]. Plasma miR-124-3p and miR-16 were considered as prognostic markers of acute stroke [28]. hsa-miR-155-5p could mediated the inflammatory response in IS [29]. The upregulating of miR-375 was shown to be involved in protective effects of calycosin on cerebral ischemia rats [30]. The upregulation of miR-146a was shown to play an important role in the neuroprotective effect of the combination therapy for acute stroke. These indicated us that the more E-CKs one miRNA regulated, the more likely it is involved in stroke related processes.

3.3   E-CK Network

All the E-CKs were mapped to the human protein-protein interaction network downloaded from HPRD database. Only interactions between two E-CKs were kept. A weighted network containing 90 E-CKs as nodes and 77 edges between them was constructed. The nodes were divided into 7 groups according to their differential expressed patterns on gene level as shown in Table 3. Two E-CKs was involved in the patterns with 'Recovery related' as the only character. Interleukin-16 (IL-16) is the only E-CKs with the differential expressed pattern 'Subacute Chronic vs. Health (Recovery related)'. This pro-inflammatory cytokine was proved to be a key element in the ischemic cascade after cerebral ischemia and its polymorphism was also validated to be associated with an increased risk of ischemic stroke [31]. Angiotensin-1-converting enzyme (ACE) is the cytokine differential expressed only between chronic stage and health condition. One study found that the deletion of ACE was common in Egyptian non-cardioembolic ischemic stroke patients [32]. All the other E-CKs were shown to have dual immune characters and the percentage of E-CKs involved in stroke related biological procedures were presented in Table 3. Interestingly, all the two E-CKs (IL18BP, PTPRC) in the chronic stage related pattern named 'Subacute vs. Chronic,' were not validated by literature currently. However, the protein encoded by IL18BP was constitutively expressed and secreted in mononuclear cells, and functioned as an inhibitor of IL18, which is the pro-inflammatory cytokine. The protein encoded by PTPRC was shown to suppress JAK kinases, and thus functions as a regulator of cytokine receptor signaling. These indicated us that IL18BP may be a potential treatment target especially in chronic stage which may help improve the recovery of stroke greatly in the future.

Table 3. Percentages of validated relationships between E-CKs and stroke.

Character	Differential expressed pattern	Percentage of stroke-related E-CKs
Dual	Acute vs. Subacute vs. Chronic Subacute vs. Health	72.00%
Dual	Acute vs. Subacute vs. Chronic Acute, Subacute vs. Health	63.64%
Dual	Subacute vs. Chronic Acute, Subacute vs. Health	60.00%
Dual	Acute vs. Subacute Acute vs. Health	31.03%
Process related	Subacute vs. Chronic	0.00%
Recovery related	Subacute, Chronic vs. Health	100.00%

4   Sources of Funding

This study was funded by the Basic Research Program of Shenzhen [JCYJ20160229203627477], the National 863 Project of China [SS2015AA020109], and the Science and Technology Planning Project of Guangdong Province [2015B010129012], and the Science and Technology Service Network Plan (STS plan) Project of Chinese Academy of Sciences – Hefei [KFJ-SW-STS-161].

References

1. Jiang, Y., Zhu, W., Zhu, J., et al.: Feasibility of delivering mesenchymal stem cells via catheter to the proximal end of the lesion artery in patients with stroke in the territory of the middle cerebral artery. Cell Transplant. **22**(12), 2291–2298 (2013)
2. Lees, K.R., Bluhmki, E., von Kummer, R., et al.: Time to treatment with intravenous alteplase and outcome in stroke: an updated pooled analysis of ECASS, ATLANTIS, NINDS, and EPITHET trials. Lancet **375**(9727), 1695–1703 (2010)
3. Fonarow, G.C., Smith, E.E., Saver, J.L., et al.: Timeliness of tissue-type plasminogen activator therapy in acute ischemic stroke: patient characteristics, hospital factors, and outcomes associated with door-to-needle times within 60 minutes. Circulation **123**(7), 750–758 (2011)
4. Lo, E.H.: Degeneration and repair in central nervous system disease. Nat. Med. **16**, 1205–1209 (2010)
5. Morancho, A., Rosell, A., Garcia-Bonilla, L., et al.: Metalloproteinase and stroke infarct size: role for anti-inflammatory treatment? Ann. N. Y. Acad. Sci. **1207**, 123–133 (2010)
6. Xu, X., Jiang, Y.: The Yin and Yang of innate immunity in stroke. Biomed. Res. Int. **2014**, 807978 (2014)
7. Shichita, T., Ago, T., Kamouchi, M., et al.: Novel therapeutic strategies targeting innate immune responses and early inflammation after stroke. J. Neurochem. **123**(supplement 2), 29–38 (2012)
8. Banwell, V., Sena, E.S., Macleod, M.R.: Systematic review and stratified meta-analysis of the efficacy of interleukin-1 receptor antagonist in animal models of stroke. J. Stroke Cerebrovasc. Dis. **18**(4), 269–276 (2009)
9. Gertz, K., Kronenberg, G., Kälin, R.E., et al.: Essential role of interleukin-6 in post-stroke angiogenesis. Brain J. Neurol. **135**(6), 1964–1980 (2012)
10. Zeng, L., Wang, Y., Liu, J., et al.: Pro-inflammatory cytokine network in peripheral inflammation response to cerebral ischemia. Neurosci. Lett. **548**, 4–9 (2013)
11. Cure, M.C., Tufekci, A., Cure, E., et al.: Low-density lipoprotein subfraction, carotid artery intima-media thickness, nitric oxide, and tumor necrosis factor alpha are associated with newly diagnosed ischemic stroke. Ann. Indian Acad. Neurol. **16**(4), 498–503 (2013)
12. Maddahi, A., Kruse, L.S., Chen, Q.W., et al.: The role of tumor necrosis factor-α and TNF-α receptors in cerebral arteries following cerebral ischemia in rat. J. Neuroinflammation **8**, 107 (2011)
13. Yingying, W., Yunpeng, C.: A survey on database resources for microRNA-disease relationships. Brief Funct. Genomics **16**(3), 146–151 (2017)
14. Yingying, W., Yunpeng, C.: Obtaining human ischemic stroke gene expression biomarkers from animal models: a cross-species validation study. Sci Rep. **6**, 29693 (2016)
15. Jing, L., Yunpeng, Z., Yingying, W., et al.: Functional combination strategy for prioritization of human miRNA target. Gene **533**(1), 132–141 (2014)
16. Yingying, W., Lei, D., Xia, L., et al.: Functional homogeneity in microRNA target heterogeneity - a new sight into human microRNomics. OMICS J. Integr. Biol. **15**(1-2), 25–35 (2011)
17. Yingying, W., Yunpeng, C.: A network-based analysis of ischemic stroke using parallel microRNA-mRNA expression profiles. In: GlobalSIP14-Workshop on Genomic Signal Processing and Statistics. Atlanta, Georgia, USA, 03–05 December 2014
18. Barrett, T., Wilhite, S.E., Ledoux, P., et al.: NCBI GEO: archive for functional genomics data sets–update. Nucleic Acids Res. **41**, D991–D995 (2013)

19. Stamova, B., Jickling, G.C., Ander, B.P., et al.: Gene expression in peripheral immune cells following cardioembolic stroke is sexually dimorphic. PLoS ONE **9**, e102550 (2014)

20. Barr, T.L., VanGilder, R., Rellick, S., et al.: A genomic profile of the immune response to stroke with implications for stroke recovery. Biol. Res. Nurs. **17**, 248–256 (2015)

21. Krug, T., Gabriel, J.P., Taipa, R., et al.: TTC7B emerges as a novel risk factor for ischemic stroke through the convergence of several genome-wide approaches. J. Cereb. Blood Flow Metab. **32**, 1061–1072 (2012)

22. Fagan, S.C., Hess, D.C., Hohnadel, E.J., et al.: Targets for vascular protection after acute ischemic stroke. Stroke **35**(9), 2220–2225 (2004)

23. Subramanian, A., Tamayo, P., Mootha, V.K., et al.: Gene set enrichment analysis: a knowledge-based approach for interpreting genome-wide expression profiles. Proc. Natl. Acad. Sci. USA **102**(43), 15545–15550 (2005)

24. Keshava Prasad, T.S., Goel, R., Kandasamy, K., et al.: Human protein reference database–2009 update. Nucleic Acids Res. **37**, D767–D772 (2009)

25. Chou, C.H., Chang, N.W., Shrestha, S., et al.: miRTarBase 2016: updates to the experimentally validated miRNA-target interactions database. Nucleic Acids Res. **44**, D239–D247 (2016)

26. Liu, F.J., Kaur, P., Karolina, D.S., et al.: MiR-335 Regulates Hif-1α to reduce cell death in both mouse cell line and rat ischemic models. PLoS ONE **10**(6), e0128432 (2015)

27. Zhang, H., Liu, L., Hu, J., et al.: MicroRNA regulatory network revealing the mechanism of inflammation in atrial fibrillation. Med. Sci. Monit. **14**(21), 3505–3513 (2015)

28. Rainer, T.H., Leung, L.Y., Chan, C.P., et al.: Plasma miR-124-3p and miR-16 concentrations as prognostic markers in acute stroke. Clin. Biochem. **49**(9), 663–668 (2016)

29. Wen, Y., Zhang, X., Dong, L., et al.: Acetylbritannilactone modulates MicroRNA-155-Mediated inflammatory response in ischemic cerebral tissues. Mol. Med. **18**(21), 197–209 (2015)

30. Wang, Y., Dong, X., Li, Z., et al.: Downregulated RASD1 and upregulated miR-375 are involved in protective effects of calycosin on cerebral ischemia/reperfusion rats. J. Neurol. Sci. **339**(1–2), 144–148 (2014)

31. Liu, X.L., Du, J.Z., Zhou, Y.M., et al.: Interleukin-16 polymorphism is associated with an increased risk of ischemic stroke. Mediators Inflamm. **2013**, Article ID 564750 (2013)

32. Mostafa, M.A., El-Nabiel, L.M., Fahmy, N.A., et al.: ACE gene in Egyptian ischemic stroke patients. J. Stroke Cerebrovasc. Dis. **25**(9), 2167–2171 (2016)

Multidimensional Analysis Framework on Massive Data of Observations of Daily Living

Jianhua Lu[1][(✉)], Baili Zhang[1], Xueyan Wang[1], and Ningyun Lu[2]

[1] Southeast University, Nanjing, China
lujianhua@seu.edu.cn
[2] Nanjing University of Aeronautics and Astronautics, Nanjing, China

Abstract. Observations of daily living (ODLs) are cues that people attend to in the course of their everyday life, that inform them about their health. In order to better understand the ODLs, we propose a set of innovative multi-dimensional analysis concepts and methods. Firstly, the ODLs are organized as directed graphs according the "observation-property" relationships and the chronological order of observations, which represents all the information in a flexible way; Secondly, a novel concept, the structure dimension, is proposed to integrate into the traditional multidimensional analysis framework. From the structure dimension that consists of three granularities, vertices, edges and subgraphs, one can get a clearer view of the ODLs; Finally, the hierarchy of ODLs Cube is introduced, and the semantics of OLAP operations, Roll-up, Drill-down and Slice/dice, are redefined to accommodate the structure dimension. The proposed structure dimension and ODLs cube are effective for multidimensional analysis of ODLs.

Keywords: ODLs · Multidimensional analysis · OLAP · Graph cube

1 Introduction

Observations of Daily Living (ODLs) provide a detailed picture of one's daily experiences, from which we could discover knowledge about health status, living styles and other information [1, 2]. The ODLs of a certain individual are composed of a sequence of observations with one observation subject and several properties.

As the amount of ODLs is continuously increasing, it is critical to develop effective tools of data analyzing to answer questions about what is endangering your health or what could we do to improve our living happiness. OLAP can analyze data in different dimensions and hierarchies. However, it's not effective or efficient in this certain scenario of ODLs analysis for the traditional OLAP tools that are based on RDBMSs. The reason lies in the multiple joins among large tables that introduced by many queries we might ask.

Since the ODLs are ubiquitous and heterogeneous, it is not a good idea of using RDMBSs as storage and management tools. In this paper we propose a graph model of ODLs based on the heterogeneous information network, and introduce an innovative multidimensional analysis framework. Our contributions can be summarized as follows:

© Springer International Publishing AG 2017
S. Siuly et al. (Eds.): HIS 2017, LNCS 10594, pp. 121–127, 2017.
https://doi.org/10.1007/978-3-319-69182-4_13

- The model of ODLs network is proposed, in which all the information of ODLs are organized into a heterogeneous network, which can represent all the related information in a flexible way.
- Based on the ODLs network, the concept of Structure Dimension is defined. From the structure dimensions, the graph structures are effectively integrated into the OLAP framework. The aggregating methods of structure dimension are also introduced.
- A graph cube model is proposed based on the ODLs network and structure dimensions, the cube hierarchy and the semantics of OLAP operations including Roll-up, Drill-down and Slice/dice are introduced as well.

The remainder of the paper is organized as follows. Related works are introduced in Sect. 2. The ODLs network is presented in Sect. 3. The concept of structure dimensions, the ODLs Cube hierarchy, and the redefined OLAP operations are introduced in Sect. 4. Section 5 summaries the entire work.

2   Related Works

Chen et al. proposed the concept of Graph OLAP the first time [5]. However, there was no overview of the Graph OLAP framework. Li et al. introduced double star model [6] including the information dimension aggregation algorithm and the topological dimension aggregation algorithm, but the application scenario was relatively simple. Zhao et al. [7] proposed Graph Cube model based on multi-dimensional network, which combined the data cube concept to lead cuboid query of graph data. But Graph Cube model can only be applied into homogeneous networks. In addition, there are some research works in particular areas and cannot handle ODLs easily, such as the works in analyzing social networks or knowledge networks presented by Yin et al. [8], Denis et al. [9], Wang et al. [10], Lilia Hannachi et al. [11], Andreas Weiler et al. [12], Qiang Qu et al. [13] and Wararat Jakawat et al. [14].

3   ODLs Network

An observation is a picture or a description of an event in daily living, records the behaviors or the states of people in a certain environment, while the states include both physiological and psychological states. It contains a core subject and some related information/properties. Multiple observations are organized as a directed graph. We define observation and ODLs Network as follows.

Definition 1 (Observation). An observation is presented as $O = <C, P>$, where C is a subject and P is a set of properties of C.

Definition 2 (ODLs Network). An ODLs network is a graph $N = (V,E,T,R_S,R_A)$, where V is a set of vertices that correspond to observation subjects and properties; $E \subseteq V \times V$ is the set of arcs representing the chronological order between observations (noted as R_S) and "observation-property" relationships (noted as R_A); T is a set of vertex types, there exists one type of vertices (of type *C*) are core vertices, i.e. observation subjects, while the others are properties.

4   Structure Dimensions and ODLs Cube

Dimension lays the foundation of OLAP [5, 6] and provides the possible perspectives for the analysis, which divides the data into different groups and constructs the cuboid lattices.

ODLs networks consist of various type of vertices, "observation-property" relationships and chronological order of observations. We categorize the structure features into vertex dimension, edge dimension and subgraph dimension.

4.1   ODLs Cube

Given an ODLs network *N*, the graph cube, ODLs Cube is established by constructing all the possible aggregate graphs with all the structure dimensions, and connecting them together according to the dimension hierarchy. The ODLs Cube consists of four parts: vertex dimension sub-cube, edge dimension sub-cube, subgraph dimension sub-cube and the base data graph.

Figure 1 shows the hierarchy of an ODLs Cube. The vertex dimension sub-cube contains all the vertex aggregate graphs with all the content granularities; the edge dimension sub-cube and the subgraph dimension sub-cube consist of all the aggregate graphs in each dimension as well. All the sub-cubes are built based on the base data, i.e. ODLs network. Edge dimensions have additional "observation-property" relationships compare to vertex dimensions; while subgraph dimensions have extra "observation-observation" orders. From subgraph dimension, the analysis procedure can roll-up to vertex dimension or edge dimension, and from edge dimension we can roll-up to vertex dimension. The drill-down operations go with the reverse directions. We will introduce

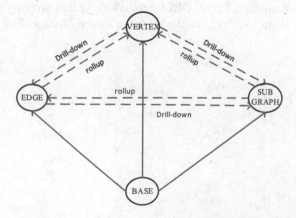

Fig. 1. The structural hierarchy of ODL cube

the detailed definitions of structure dimension, intra-dimension hierarchy and inter-dimension hierarchy respectively in the following subsections.

4.2   Structure Dimension and ODLs Cube Hierarchy

Definition 3 (Vertex Dimension). Given $N = (V, E, T, R_S, R_A)$, its vertex dimension is a subset of V with specified criteria.

Through vertex dimension, we can view ODLs networks from the vertex angle without considering arcs. Some vertices may have contents that can be grouped by different granularities, e.g. time has "year-> month-> week-> day-> hour" granularities. We allow aggregating vertices by a sequence of predefined granularities ($T < g_1$, g_2, ..., $g_k >$). Figure 2 shows the lattice of vertex dimension. Given an ODLs network, each aggregation graph is called a cuboid. In Fig. 2, cuboid "ALL" is the total number of vertices, "$T_i(ALL)$" is the vertex number of type T_i, and "(g_{ij})" is the vertex number of type T_i with granularity $T_i(g_j)$. From cuboid "ALL", we can drill-down to a specified vertex type, and down further to cuboids with smaller content granularities. Roll-up operations are the reverse.

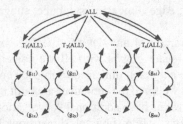

Fig. 2. The lattice of vertex dimension

Definition 4 (Edge Dimension). Given $N = (V, E, T, R_S, R_A)$, its edge dimension is a subset of R_A with specified criteria.

Through edge dimension, we can view ODLs networks from the angle of "observation-property" relationships. For an ODLs network N with m property types, its edge aggregate graphs is up to 2^m. Figure 3 shows the lattice of edge dimension. Cuboid

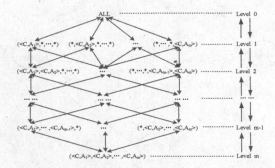

Fig. 3. The Intra-group OLAP on edge dimension

"*ALL*" aggregates the core vertices (observation subjects) with no observation property specified, from which we can drill-down to analyze the observations with one property specified, and then drill further down to observations with multiple properties specified. The lattice hierarchy is defined by the number of given properties. At the bottom of the lattice there are observations with all properties specified.

Definition 5 (Subgraph Dimension). Given $N = (V, E, T, R_S, R_A)$, its subgraph dimension is denoted as $G_s \times A$, where $G_s \subset R_S$ and $A = T - \{C\}$.

Subgraph dimension is the most complex dimension, through which we can view ODLs networks from the angle of observation-observation order relationships as well as the "observation-property" relationships. Figure 4 shows the sub-cube hierarchy of subgraph dimension. The upmost cuboids are statistics about single observations (i.e. vertices of type *C*), from which we can drill down to the cuboids with two consecutive observations, and then drill further down to the ones with longer observation sequences. In Fig. 4, P means the length of observation sequence and an edge dimension lattice is assigned to each core vertex in the sequence to express the "observation-property" constraints.

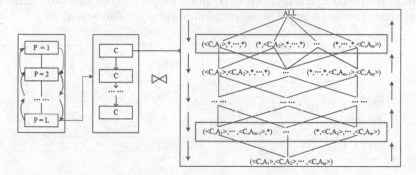

Fig. 4. The Intra-group OLAP on subgraph dimension

As we have seen, the Roll-up and Drill-down operations can be performed easily between cuboids of consecutive levels within vertex dimension, edge dimension and subgraph dimension. It's relatively easy to implement Slice/Dice operations by finding the required sub-cubes based on the specified structure dimensions. Due to the space limit, the details are not introduced.

From Fig. 1, we know there are connections between any two sub-cubes. Figure 5 shows the connections between vertex dimension and edge dimension. We can Drill-down from vertex dimension to edge dimension by selecting one core vertex cuboid and multiple property vertex cuboids.

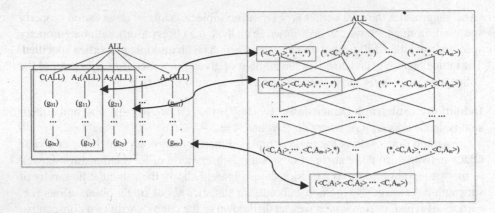

Fig. 5. Inter-dimension connections between vertex-edge dimensions

Figure 6 shows the connections between vertex dimension and subgraph dimension. The Drill-down operations are from vertex dimension to subgraph dimension by selecting multiple core vertex cuboids and multiple property vertex cuboids. The number of core vertex cuboids selected is the level within subgraph dimension.

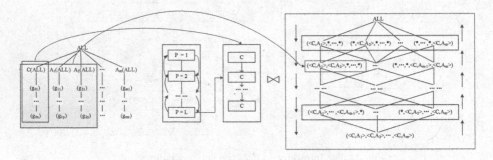

Fig. 6. Inter-dimension connections between vertex-subgraph dimensions

The connections between edge dimension and subgraph dimension are relatively straightforward. A cuboid of edge dimension is actually a length one cuboid of subgraph dimension. So, by specifying multiple cuboids of edge dimension, we can easily drill down to cuboids of subgraph dimension.

For the above three cases, the Roll-ups are the reverse of corresponding Drill-downs. This paper does not cover the details due to the space limit.

5   Conclusions and Future Works

In this paper, we studied multidimensional analysis technologies on ODLs for self-management and personal decision support. We first introduced ODLs network to model ODLs, in which observations and their properties can all be involved into structural features, and the chronological orders of observations were preserved as well. We then proposed the Structure Dimension that provided overview of ODLs from each structural perspective. We also introduced the concept and hierarchy of the ODLs Cube, and the semantics of OLAP operations, Roll-up, Drill-down and Slice/dice, are redefined as well. By using the proposed concepts and algorithms, we implemented a graph-based multidimensional analysis prototype system that is not included in this paper due to the space limit. Various examples show its effectiveness.

As for the future works, we think the system performance and the algorithm optimization issues are critical. The tools for migrating data from RDBMSs to the proposed framework are also required. And we look forward to extending the framework to other graph models.

References

1. Backonja, U., et al.: Observations of daily living: putting the "personal" in personal health records. In: NI 2012: Proceedings of the 11th International Congress on Nursing Informatics, vol. 2012. American Medical Informatics Association (2012)
2. Wolf, G.: The data-driven life. The New York Times **28**, 2010 (2010)
3. Harinarayan, V., Rajaraman, A., Ullman, J.D.: Implementing data cubes efficiently. ACM SIGMOD Rec. **25**(2), 205–216 (1996)
4. Gray, J., et al.: Data cube: a relational aggregation operator generalizing group-by, cross-tab, and sub-totals. Data Min. Knowl. Disc. **1**(1), 29–53 (1997)
5. Chen, C., et al.: Graph OLAP: towards online analytical processing on graphs. In: Proceeding of the Eighth IEEE International Conference on Data Mining (2008)
6. Li, C., et al.: Modeling, design and implementation of graph OLAPing. J. Softw. **22**(2), 258–268 (2011)
7. Zhao, P., et al.: Graph cube: on warehousing and OLAP multidimensional networks. In: Proceeding of the 2011 ACM SIGMOD International Conference on Management of Data (2011)
8. Yin, M., Bin, W., Zeng, Z.: HMGraph OLAP: a novel framework for multi-dimensional heterogeneous network analysis. In: Proceeding of the 15th International Workshop on Data Warehousing and OLAP (2012)
9. Denis, B., Ghrab, A., Skhiri, S.: A distributed approach for graph-oriented multidimensional analysis. In: Proceeding of 2013 IEEE International Conference on Big Data (2013)
10. Wang, Z., et al.: Pagrol: parallel graph OLAP over large-scale attributed graphs. In: ICDE 2014 (2014)
11. Hannachi, L., et al.: Social microblogging cube. In: Proceeding of the 16th International Workshop on Data Warehousing and OLAP (2013)
12. Rehman, N.U., Weiler, A., Scholl, M.H.: OLAPing social media: the case of Twitter. In: Proceeding of the 2013 IEEE/ACM International Conference on Advances in Social Networks Analysis and Mining (2013)
13. Qu, Q., et al.: Efficient topological OLAP on information networks. In: Database Systems for Advanced Applications (2011)
14. Jakawat, W., Favre, C., Loudcher, S.: OLAP on information networks: a new framework for dealing with bibliographic data. In: Catania, B., et al. (eds.) New Trends in Databases and Information Systems. Advances in Intelligent Systems and Computing, vol. 241, pp. 361–370. Springer, Cham (2014). doi:10.1007/978-3-319-01863-8_38
15. Brennan, P.F., Casper, G.: Observing health in everyday living: ODLs and the care-between-the-care. Pers. Ubiquit. Comput. **19**(1), 3–8 (2015)

Numerical Modeling of the Internal Temperature in the Mammary Gland

M.V. Polyakov[1]([⊠]), A.V. Khoperskov[1]([⊠]), and T.V. Zamechnic[2]([⊠])

[1] Volgograd State University, Volgograd, Russia
{m.v.polyakov,khoperskov}@volsu.ru
[2] Volgograd State Medical University, Volgograd, Russia
tvzamechnic.61@mail.ru

Abstract. The microwave thermometry method for the diagnosis of breast cancer is based on an analysis of the internal temperature distribution. This paper is devoted to the construction of a mathematical model for increasing the accuracy of measuring the internal temperature of mammary glands, which are regarded as a complex combination of several components, such as fat tissue, muscle tissue, milk lobules, skin, blood flows, tumor tissue. Each of these biocomponents is determined by its own set of physical parameters. Our numerical model is designed to calculate the spatial distributions of the electric microwave field and the temperature inside the biological tissue. We compare the numerical simulations results to the real medical measurements of the internal temperature.

1 Introduction

The method of microwave thermometry (RTM) has become significant recently for oncological diagnostics [1,4,14,15]. This method allows to conduct surveys frequently and without any harm to health [13]. The RTM is based on measuring the temperature inside the biological tissue at various points [2,3,5,11]. Then the received data is subject to intellectual analysis to assist doctor with the diagnosis. Using the method of combined thermography, we consistently measure temperatures at 9 different points of the female breast [10,11]. Instrumental internal and surface temperatures of tissues are determined by the intensity of their thermal radiation in the microwave and infrared ranges, respectively. Body temperature distribution is an important criterion in the diagnosis of diseases [11,13] because it characterizes a person's functional state. Tumors of the breast cause relatively high heat emission at an early stage, which leads to a local increase in the temperature of the tissues.

To increase the efficiency of diagnosis of oncological disease we study the results of a series of computer experiments on calculation the internal temperature in the microwave range with the radiothermometry method. An important problem of modeling biological tissues is the variability of individual physical characteristics of biological tissue of different people. We use the model that is

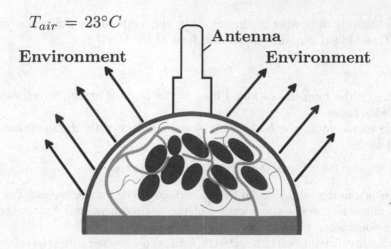

Fig. 1. The general scheme of our model

based on the numerical integration of Maxwell's equations and heat equation for multicomponent biological tissue.

The novelty of our approach is based on multifaceted computational models that take into account the multicomponent properties of biological tissues and their complex spatial structure. As a rule, the heat sources associated with the blood flow are considered in the capillary approximation, when the heat release is evenly distributed over the volume of the tissue [8,14]. Our model contains a branched system of blood vessels of different diameters, and the heat release is not uniform.

The complex spatial structure of a mammary gland and small-scale inhomogeneity (Fig. 1) require the use of unstructured numerical grids for calculating electric and temperature fields. Typical sizes of numerical cells are approximately 0.02–0.1 mm.

2 Mathematical Model

Computer modeling is based on the numerical solving of the heat equation for biological tissue [2,8,10,14]:

$$\rho(\mathbf{r})c_p(\mathbf{r})\frac{\partial T_{mod}}{\partial t}(\mathbf{r},t) = \nabla(\delta(\mathbf{r})\nabla T_{mod}(\mathbf{r},t))$$

$$+ Q_{bl}(\mathbf{r},t) + Q_{met}(\mathbf{r},t) - Q_{rad}(\mathbf{r},t),$$

(1)

where ρ is the volume density of tissue, $c_p(\mathbf{r})$ is the specific heat of material, T_{mod} is the simulated temperature, Q_{bl} is the heat source from blood vessels, Q_{met} is the heat source from metabolic processes in biological tissues, Q_{rad} is radiation cooling, δ is the coefficient of thermal conductivity, $\nabla = \left\{\dfrac{\partial}{\partial x}, \dfrac{\partial}{\partial y}, \dfrac{\partial}{\partial z}\right\}$ is the nabla operator.

The intensity of heating is determined by the temperature difference between tissue T and blood T_{bl}, and the specific heat of the blood $c_{p,b}$

$$Q_{bl} = -\rho\rho_{bl}c_{p,b}\omega_{bl}(T - T_{bl}), \tag{2}$$

where ω_{bl} is the intensity of blood flow in the heating region, which can vary over a wide range.

Heat exchange at the biological tissue boundary with the environment is defined as

$$(\mathbf{n}\nabla T) = \frac{h_{air}}{\delta(\mathbf{r})}\left[T(\mathbf{r}) - T_{air}\right], \tag{3}$$

where $\mathbf{n}$ is a unit vector normal to the surface of the female breast. The value of T_{air} characterizes the temperature of the environment and h_{air} is the heat transfer coefficient.

Stationary distribution of the electric field is constructed using the calculation for the establishment and solving the nonstationary Maxwell's equations:

$$\frac{\partial \mathbf{B}}{\partial t} + \text{rot}(\mathbf{E}) = 0, \tag{4}$$

$$\frac{\partial \mathbf{D}}{\partial t} - \text{rot}(\mathbf{H}) = 0, \tag{5}$$

$$\mathbf{B} = \mu(\mathbf{r})\mathbf{H}, \quad \mathbf{D} = \varepsilon(\mathbf{r})\mathbf{E}. \tag{6}$$

Antenna allows to measure thermal radiation in the frequency range $f_{min} \leq f \leq f_{max}$. Biological tissue has an inhomogeneous temperature. This method gives a weighted average temperature T_{int} in the region V_0 [7]. The error of the method is due to the noise temperature of the receiver T_{noise}, the mismatch effects in the antenna $s(f)$, the environmental effect T_{env}. The internal temperature is determined by the integral representation [12,14]:

$$T_{int} = \int_{\Delta f}\left[(1 - |s(f)|^2)\left(\int_V W(\mathbf{r},f)\,T_{mod}(\mathbf{r})\,dV + T_{env}\right) + |s(f)|^2 T_{noise}\right]df \tag{7}$$

with weighting function

$$W(\mathbf{r},f) = \frac{F(\mathbf{r},f)}{\int_V F(\mathbf{r},f)\,dV}, \quad \int_V W(\mathbf{r},f)\,dV = 1, \tag{8}$$

$$F(\mathbf{r},f) = \frac{1}{2}\sigma(\mathbf{r},f)\,|E(\mathbf{r},f)|^2. \tag{9}$$

The value W according to the principle of reciprocity coincides with the density of the power F (W/m^3) and depends on the electrical conductivity of σ and electric field $\mathbf{E}$ inside a certain volume V. Efficiency of temperature T_{int} measurementby a radiometer strongly depends on electromagnetic interference T_{noise}, which requires proper shielding.

The receiving antenna is the key element of the radiothermometer.

An important task is to achieve a low level of mismatch s between the antenna and biotissue. The antenna should ensure a deep penetration into the biotissue. It depends on the ratio of energy from brown fat tissue to total power.

3   Results of Computer Modeling

The input data for modeling are the physical parameters of the biocomponent (Table 1).

The T_{mod} calculation is performed using the Comsol Multiphysics version 4.3 a [6]. The E calculation is performed using the CST Microwave Studio

Table 1. Physical parameters of components [10]

	Skin	Mammary gland	Connective tissue	Bloodstream
Dielectric permeability, ε	53.5–57.2	5.1–5.9	44.2–48.1	1.54–1.96
Electric conduction, σ (1/Ohm)	0.92–1.31	0.03–0.09	2.19–2.68	45.8–48.2
Resistivity, $\mathcal{R}$ (Ohm·m)	53.1–56.9	13.9–15.7	1.31–1.74	1.22–1.7

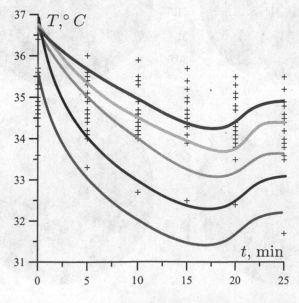

Fig. 2. Comparison of the results of numerical experiments (color lines) with the data of real medical measurements (+) (Color figure online)

simulation package [9]. Calculation of the deep temperature is carried out with the mathematical package Scilab.

The mechanism of adaptation of a living organism to environmental conditions deserves special attention. Physiological adaptation is associated with the regulation of the physiological functions of the organism. Thermoregulation is the ability of living organisms to maintain the temperature of their body at a constant level or to change it within certain limits.

We measure 20 patients for 25 min with an interval of 5 min. Most medical measurements have fully confirmed the thermoregulation process. We found a trend. The temperature starts to increase from 20th minute after the decrease. We consider this process in our model. The amount of heat that gives blood streams to biological tissues increases from 20th minute.

We perform numerical experiments and we vary the values of physical parameters of the biocomponent in each new calculation. The results of numerical simulation are compared with the results of medical measurements (Fig. 2). We use the patient data for the left breast cancer at the point «0» [10].

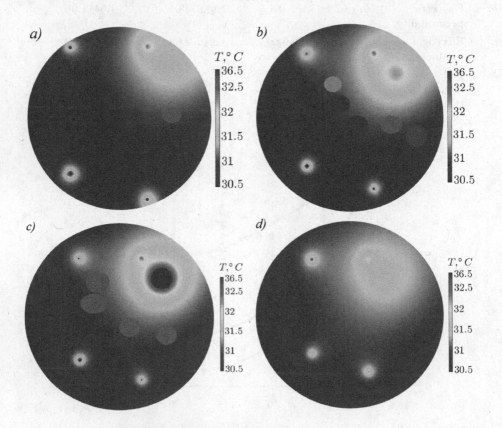

Fig. 3. Temperature map of the model with tumor $R = 0.5$ sm, at a depth 2.5 sm and (a) $z = 4$ sm, (b) $z = 3$ sm, (c) $z = 2.5$ sm, (d) $z = 2$ sm

As we see, the results of the numerical experiment are consistent with the data of medical measurements.

We constructed temperature maps for the model with a tumor based on the results of numerical experiment (Fig. 3). Strong asymmetric temperature in regions with and without a tumor is observed on the basis of this temperature map [8,11].

We carried out the computational experiments to study the dependence of temperature fields on the presence of tumor tissue in a mammary gland. Malignant neoplasms, especially in the early stages of development, have an extremely

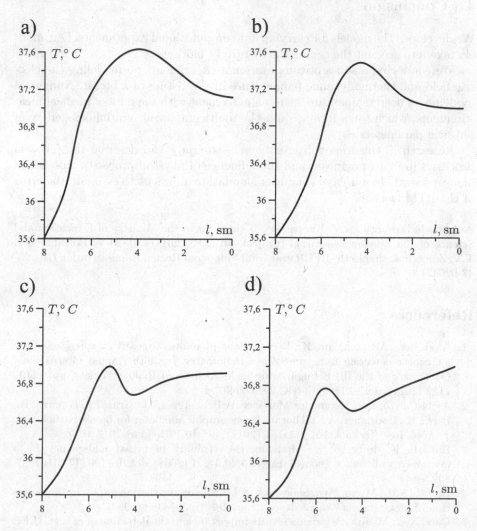

Fig. 4. Temperature distribution along the depth for tumors of various diameters D, (*a*) $D = 2\,\text{sm}$, (*b*) $D = 1.5\,\text{sm}$, (*c*) $D = 1\,\text{sm}$, (*d*) $D = 0.7\,\text{sm}$

high heat release, with respect to the remaining biological components. We examined tumors of different diameters $(D = 2\,\text{sm}, D = 1.5\,\text{sm}, D = 1\,\text{sm}, D = 0.7\,\text{sm})$.

We obtained the following results (Fig. 4). The radius of a tumor affects the temperature background inside the volume of mammary gland. The average temperature is higher, the larger the radius of the tumor. This is the main problem of diagnosis: detection of cancer at an early stage $(R < 0.5)$. A tumor of this size is difficult to detect with modern diagnostic methods.

4   Conclusion

We developed the models for carrying out computational experiments. Our models take into account the complex structure of biotissue.

We conducted a series of computational experiments on modeling the electric field and thermodynamic temperature in the tissues of a breast. Numerical modeling of deep temperature gives an agreement with the data of medical measurements, which takes into account the multicomponent and inhomogenety of physical parameters.

Research in this area will greatly help to study and describe the physical processes in living organisms and the influence of physical processes on medical measurements. In our case, computer simulation allows us to estimate the error of the RTM method.

Acknowledgments. A.V. Khoperskov is thankful to the Ministry of Education and Science of the Russian Federation (project No. 2.852.2017/4.6). M.V. Polyakov and T.V. Zamechnic thanks the RFBR grant and Volgograd Region Administration (No. 15-47-02642).

References

1. Akki, R.S., Arunachalam, K.: Breast tissue phantoms to assist compression study for cancer detection using microwave radiometry. In: 36th Annual International Conference of the IEEE Engineering in Medicine and Biology Society, pp. 1119–1122 (2014). doi:10.1109/EMBC.2014.6943791
2. Avila-Castro, I.A., Hernandez-Martinez, A.R., Estevez, M., Cruz, M., Esparza, R., Perez, R., Rodriguez, A.L.: Thorax thermographic simulator for breast pathologies. J. Appl. Res. Technol. **15**, 143–151 (2017). doi:10.1016/j.jart.2017.01.008
3. Bardati, F., Iudicello, S.: Modeling the visibility of breast malignancy by a microwave radiometer. Biomed. Eng. **55**, 214–221 (2008). doi:10.1109/TBME.2007.899354
4. Barett, A.H., Myers, P.C., Sadowsky, N.L.: Microwave thermography in the detection of breast canser. Am. J. Roentgenol. **34**(2), 365–368 (1980)
5. Carr, K.L.: Microwave radiometry: its importance to the detection of cancer. IEEE MTT **37**, 12–24 (1989)
6. Datta, A., Rakesh, V.: An Introduction to Modeling of Transport Processes: Applications to Biomedical Systems. Cambridge University Press, 503 p. (2009)

7. Foster, K.R., Cheever, E.A.: Microwave radiometry in biomedicine: a reappraisal. Bioelectromagnetics **13**(6), 567–579 (1992)
8. Gonzalez, F.J.: Thermal simulation of breast tumors. Revista Mexicana de Fisica **53**, 323–326 (2007)
9. Kurushin, A.A., Plastikov, A.N.: Design of Microwave Devices in CST Microwave Studio. MEI Press, 155 p
10. Losev, A.G., Khoperskov, A.V., Astakhov, A.S., Suleymanova, K.M.: Problems of measurement and modeling of thermal and radiation fields in biological tissues: analysis of microwave thermometry data. Sci. J. Volgograd State Univ. Math. Phys. **6**(31), 98–142 (2015). doi:10.15688/jvolsu1.2015.6.3
11. Novochadov, V.V., Shiroky, A.A., Khoperskov, A.V., Losev, A.G.: Comparative modeling the thermal transfer in tissues with volume pathological focuses and tissue engineering constructs: a pilot study. European Journal of. Mol. Biotechnol. **14**(4), 125–138 (2016). doi:10.13187/ejmb.2016.14.125
12. Polyakov, M.V., Khoperskov, A.V.: Mathematical modeling of radiation fields in biological tissues: the definition of the brightness temperature for the diagnosis. Sci. J. Volgograd State Univ. Math. Phys. **5**(36), 73–84 (2016). doi:10.15688/jvolsu1.2016.5.7
13. Shah, T.H., Siores, E., Daskalakis, C.: Non-invasive devices for early detection of breast tissue oncological abnormalities using microwave radio thermometry. In: Gali-Muhtasib, H. (eds.) Advances in Cancer Therapy. InTech, pp. 447–476 (2011). doi:10.5772/23586
14. Vesnin, S.G., Sedakin, K.M.: Development of antenna-applicator series for tissue temperature non-invasive measurement of a human. Eng. J. Sci. Innov. **11**, 1–18 (2012)
15. Vrba, J., Oppl, L., Vrbova, B.: Microwaves in medical diagnostics and treatment. In: 24th International Conference Radioelektronika, Bratislava, pp. 1–6 (2014). doi:10.1109/Radioelek.2014.6828405

Research on Multidimensional Modelling for Personal Health Record

Hao Fan[1,2(✉)], Jianping He[1], and Gang Liu[3]

[1] School of Information Management, Wuhan University, Wuhan, China
hfan@whu.edu.cn
[2] Center for Studies of Information Resources, Wuhan University, Wuhan, China
[3] School of Information Management, Central China Normal University,
Wuhan, China

Abstract. Personal Health Records (PHRs) have characteristics of continuous high speed growth and rich value, which are the prerequisite and foundation for implementing services of intelligent health care, personalized medicine, remote treatment, disease prevention and prediction, and the strong support for the hospital, health care institutions, insurance companies and other organizations to maintain personal health. PHR contents have multidimensional features such as time, region, population and role orientation, which have different semantic meaning and application value. As the fundamental element of semantic web technology architecture, ontology provides an expressive framework for reusing, sharing, representing and reasoning knowledge, and has been widely applied in modelling biological, medicine and health care fields. This paper analyzes the multidimensional features of PHRs, and investigates an approach for modelling PHRs based on current existing health record standards by using ontology modelling methods and theoretical frameworks.

Keywords: Personal Health Record · Multidimensional modelling · Ontology · HL7 · openEHR

1 Introduction

A Personal Health Record (PHR) is a health record where health data and information related to the care of a patient are maintained by the patient [1], and nowadays PHRs are extended to collect, track and share past and current health information about common people rather than patients. PHRs can contain a diverse range of data, such as laboratory test results, prescription records, allergies and adverse drug reactions, illness and hospitalization documents, medications and dosing, surgeries and other procedures, vaccination records, family history, Observations of Daily Living and so on. PHRs have characteristics of continuous high speed growth and rich value, which are the prerequisite and foundation for implementing services of intelligent health care, personalized medicine, remote treatment, disease prevention and prediction. In addition to storing health information for individuals, some PHRs provide added-value

© Springer International Publishing AG 2017
S. Siuly et al. (Eds.): HIS 2017, LNCS 10594, pp. 136–148, 2017.
https://doi.org/10.1007/978-3-319-69182-4_15

services such as drug-drug interaction checking, electronic messaging between patients and providers, managing appointments, and reminders. Thus, establishing an effective mechanism for managing PHRs is the requirement of setting up medical and health service systems and implementing the *Residents Health Action Plan*.

There are existing health records standards, i.e. the Health Level Seven (HL7) V3 Reference Information model [2] and the openEHR Reference Model [3], presenting the methods modelling clinical information. A reference model in systems, enterprise, and software engineering is an abstract framework or domain-specific ontology consisting of an interlinked set of clearly defined concepts produced by an expert or body of experts in order to encourage clear communication, which is often illustrated as a set of concepts with some indication of the relationships between the concepts. PHR contents have multidimensional features such as time, region, population and role orientation dimensions, which have different semantic meaning and application value. As the fundamental element of semantic web technology architecture, ontology provides an expressive framework for reusing, sharing, representing and reasoning knowledge, mainly dealing with interoperation of heterogeneous data, reusing and sharing in knowledge engineering, representation and abstraction. So far, ontology has been widely applied in biological science (e.g. large-scale gene ontology), publishing field (e.g. Dublin-core standard and knowledge classification ontology), medicine and health care field (e.g. cancer ontology) and culture inheritance field (e.g. museum and artist ontology), which is beneficial for information system developing and knowledge modelling in different domains.

This paper identifies the requirements for multidimensional modelling PHRs as a prerequisite for the construction of a PHR management system, and proposes an approach constructing the PHR ontology model, which is conducive to the expansion of knowledge organization application domains and contribution to the realization of PHR application values. In addition, based on the PHR ontology model, this paper establishes a specific disease domain model — hypertension PHR ontology model, which is able to provide a platform for organizing information about hypertension and provide data support for hospitals, health care institutions, insurance companies to maintain personal health by providing health care services. The hypertension PHR ontology model is the first step to establish a complete PHR ontology model.

2   Related Work

2.1   Research on Ontology-Based Modelling Techniques

In order to overcome the disadvantages of traditional knowledge modelling methods, such as classification and thesaurus, in terms of ambiguities for knowledge understanding and difficulties for knowledge association and reasoning, ontology model is introduced to the process of organizing knowledge. In recent years, the research of ontology-based information modelling and knowledge organization has become a hot topic in relevant areas, which mainly involves the ontology theory, ontology construction and application research, and has been widely used in various domains. Karshenas et al. present an ontology-based approach building information models to facilitate information exchange among different knowledge domain applications, which is based on a shared building ontology that models building domain element types and relationships. The integrated information system should be modelled using shared ontologies, and each knowledge domain adds its own element properties to the shared building ontology [4].

In the field of digital library, ontology formal models and specific functions, concepts and features have been investigated and applied, and is treated as a tool to describe the conceptual system in the level of knowledge and semantics in the process of organizing knowledge for digital libraries [5,6]. Similarly, the method of ontology-based information modelling has also been applied to the medical field. For example, Mi and Cao produce an approach systematically controlling the domain ontology through the top ontology, integrating knowledge ontologies of Chinese nasal inflammation diseases and national essential medicines, and using the integrated ontology to annotate electronic medical records and related information resources in order to construct a knowledge base in XML format [7]. Shen et al. represent, reveal and manage knowledge of image reports, by analyzing composition structures, terms and term relationships in contexts [8].

In the field of medical and health, ontologies have been widely used in health information management to improve data consistency and interoperability between systems. Under the guidance of a single ontology, a holistic ontology framework can be constructed. The PHR ontology model needs to be built to manage health information based on ontology. The construction of PHR ontology model is mainly accomplished by model requirement analysis, semantic construction, concept mapping relation and determination of index [9].

2.2 Research on Multidimensional Knowledge Organization

The multidimensional characteristics of knowledge have gradually attracted the attention of researchers. Casselman and Samson propose that knowledge has multiple dimension attributes which are beyond the explicit and implicit features, and the effectiveness of knowledge contents is varied in different dimensions. Four dimensions of knowledge are presented: *content dimension, structure dimension, time dimension* and *social-impact dimension* [10]. Goeken et al. identify the requirement for multidimensional modelling techniques of data warehouse development [11].

Knowledge contents are different from different granularities, which is also a manifestation of the multidimensional characteristics of knowledge, and researchers have tried to improve the existing knowledge organization method to carry out multidimensional perspectives. Guo et al. combine the granularity computing method with Facet-based Classification theory together to define granularity attributes and semantic relations for different users [12]. Lv et al. propose a method constructing multidimensional dynamic knowledge by using knowledge maps [13]. Xu et al. represent different knowledge through the concept and composition of knowledge-granularity, and use knowledge aggregation methods to quantify associations between knowledge and user requirements, and establish specifications for knowledge partitioning and granularity based on existing norms [14]. In addition to existing methods and specifications, researchers have tried to introduce new concepts and methods. Wang draws on Lattice theory in materials science, propose an approach using irregular knowledge lattice for flexible organization of multidimensional knowledge, which provided references for the further research of multidimensional knowledge aggregation and discovery [15]. In recent conferences of International Society for Knowledge Organization, researchers discuss issues of time influences on the Facet-based Classification framework, the epistemological meaning of time and space in classification system, the construction of multi-aspect music ontologies, etc., but rarely involve the problems such as the differences of knowledge connotation in different dimensions, according knowledge organization methods and its applications.

2.3   Research on Personal Health Record and Application

The *National Alliance for Health Information Technology* (*NAHIT*) report defines PHR as an electronic record of health-related information on an individual that conforms to nationally recognized interoperability standards and that can be drawn from multiple sources while being managed, shared, and controlled by the individual [1]. Research on PHRs mainly focus on three aspects:

(1) PHR Standards. In order to construct PHRs, the first is to develop a unified, scientific and reasonable PHR data standard. At present, data standards of PHR in China mainly include three types: *the health service basic data set standard, the health record common metadata standard,* and *the health record metadata classification code standard* [16], while in abroad mainly include: *European standard EN 13606, HL7 Clinical Document Architecture* (CDA) and *openEHR.* The HL7 CDA is a health information exchange standard between different medical applications. As an electron transmission protocol and standard of hospital data information, HL7 is also the standard of clinical medicine and management information format, and used for defining PHR data transmission [17].

(2) PHR Modelling. In the research of PHR modelling, researchers propose PHR models based on the openEHR standard [18] and XML technology [19]. openEHR is an open standard specification in health informatics that describes the management and storage, retrieval and exchange of health data in electronic health records (EHRs). In openEHR, all health data for a person is stored in a "one lifetime", vendor-independent, person-centred EHR [3]. There are also scholars integrating ontology and semantic extraction technologies into the construction of PHR knowledge bases, and putting forward the idea of ontology-based knowledge bases of health records [20].

(3) PHR Application. The research on PHR application is mostly concentrated in the management of PHRs. A PHR system is able to effectively combine personal health data, medical knowledge and software tools, to provide a basis for self health management and personalized controlling of patients [21]. For

example, PHR platforms can be applied for diabetes management [22], hypertension therapy [23], safe medication [24], and so on. In addition, the combination of PHR systems and cloud computing techniques are proposed based on the sharing characteristics of cloud computing software and hardware. Bahga and Madisetti discuss health data standards and exchange methods [25], and Zhang propose the service architecture of a cloud PHR system [26].

In summary, methods of ontology-based knowledge organization exhibit unique advantages in organizing static knowledge, which can clearly demonstrate concepts of static knowledge and relationships between concepts and be applied in various domains. This methods have been mature in theory, technology and tool aspects. In the field of health care, static knowledge refers to the regularity of disease occurrence and development, such as certain cure treatments for specific diseases, while relative knowledge is the detection of Individual blood pressure, weight and other indicators, and dynamic knowledge refers to the prevention and treatment of diseases carried out by individuals, which is varied with time and personal circumstances. The existing methods need to be further explored and strengthened to handle multi-granularity knowledge.

So far, the research on multidimensional knowledge organization is still in the initial stage, in terms of discussing the multidimensional characteristics and several knowledge organization methods. The application and empirical research of multidimensional knowledge organization in specific domains are rarely involved. Meanwhile, the research of PHRs mainly focuses on establishing, managing and maintaining data standards, where most of them are at the stage of exploration and conception. On the one hand, the promotion and popularization of PHRs needs to be strengthened. On the other hand, it would be a new research trend of managing and utilizing PHRs from the perspective of knowledge organization, especially in the filed of multidimensional knowledge.

3   Multidimensional Features of Personal Health Record

The *Basic Framework and Data Standard of Health Archives (on Trial)*, promulgated by the Ministry of Health in 2009, indicates that health record data has features of multi-channel source, multi-view description and multi-aspect sharing. As a kind of knowledge resources, PHRs have the characteristics of diversification in source structures, semantic dimensions and service objects.

(1) A PHR is a collection of health data from different data collection terminals, including physical examination data, medical data, personal daily monitoring data, etc. PHR and Electronic Health Record (EHR) are not the same in many aspects, although the two are related to the collection of data. In EHR the hospital or the practitioner creates and has control over all the documents, while in PHR it is the individual. PHR helps a person to be more alert in their health care, and EHR helps a practitioner to give the best treatment and also to reduce errors while proving health care to patients.

(2) A PHR can be used to analyze and organize the knowledge connotation from the aspects of time, region and population. For example, coal mine workers

are at high risk of pneumoconiosis, and their regular lung physical examination data should be focused on monitoring. Also, the human body have different blood pressure reference standards in terms of body weight, age, family history and even day and night times.

(3) A PHR can be divided into different service objects according to different business systems, life periods and administrative regions, and the knowledge content is also specifically organized via analyzing relationships between data items and service objects. A PHR contains information about the symptoms, medicines taken, special diets, exercise programs and information of home monitoring devices. It also includes information like allergies, illnesses, hospitalisations, surgeries, vaccinations and lab results. Only specific information requires specific services, and only the information need related to this service is relevant. Furthermore, the information need is also affected by the role of the service user.

According to the above, times, regions and populations are well-known challenging modelling problems in PHRs, which is a by-produce of the investigation, intervention and observation processes in a PHR management system, such as time of measurement, region of risk and population of tendency. In addition, different role and service objects, e.g. individuals, hospitals, practitioners, and insurance companies, have different requirements of PHR contents. Thus, we declare that PHRs have multidimensional features in terms of time, region, population and role orientation, which urgently require to be concretely modelled.

4   Modelling Personal Health Record

The PHR reference model is concerned with the semantics of information that needs to be stored and processed in a PHR management system, as a set of concepts with some indication of the relationships between the concepts. It is proposed for regulating the logic framework of PHR data, and used for the data collection and information sharing of health archives. Although there is no specific statement of the contents of a reference model should be included, it is generally considered to be consist of a taxonomy of terms, concepts and definitions, logic and functional components, object models, data types, communication interfaces, and so on. In this paper, based on the HL3 V3 RIM and openEHR RM, we mainly consider the object model in the ontology level of PHRs in term of handling the multidimensional features.

4.1   The HL7 V3 Reference Information Model

The HL7 Reference Information Model (RIM) is a static model of health and health care information as viewed within the scope of HL7 standards development activities, which is an object mode and a pictorial representation of the HL7 clinical data (domains) and identifies the life cycle that a message or groups of related messages will carry [2]. The RIM is comprised of six back-bone classes at the abstract level, as shown in Fig. 1, including Entity, Role, RoleLink, Participation, Act and ActRelationship classes. Where Entity class represents the physical

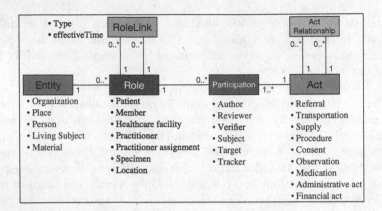

Fig. 1. The HL7 V3 RIM architecture

things and beings that are of interest to, and take part in health care; Act class represents the actions that are executed and must be documented as health care is managed and provided; ActRelationship class represents the binding of one act to another, such as the relationship between an order for an observation and the observation event as it occurs; Role class establishes the roles that entities play as they participate in health care acts; RoleLink class represents relationships between individual roles; Participation class expresses the context for an act in terms such as who performed it, for whom it was done, where it was done, etc.;

However, the RIM architecture provides a static view of the information needs of HL7 V3 standards, and can not be directly implemented for dynamically modelling the information of a health record management system, such as handling the time, region and population dimension of the records.

4.2   The OpenEHR Information Model

The abstract specifications of the openEHR architecture [3] consist of packages of Reference Model (RM), Service Model (SM) and Archetype Model (AM), which provides an approach to modelling information, services and domain knowledge in healthcare systems. The RM package, as the bottom-most layers in the architecture, provides identifiers, access to knowledge resources, data types and structures, versioning semantics and various common design patterns that can be reused ubiquitously in the upper layers of the RM, and equally in the AM and SM packages. It is composed of nine components, i.e. the Support, Data Types, Data Structures, Common, Security, EHR, EHR Extract, Integration and Demographics Information Model (IM), in which the ERH IM defines a logical EHR information architecture providing the containment and context semantics of the key concepts of health records, such as EHR, COMPOSITION, SECTION, and ENTRY. Figure 2 is the overview of the ERH Information Model [3].

The main data of the EHR is modelled as the concept of COMPOSITION, in which the ENTRY classes are the most important in the EHR IM, since they

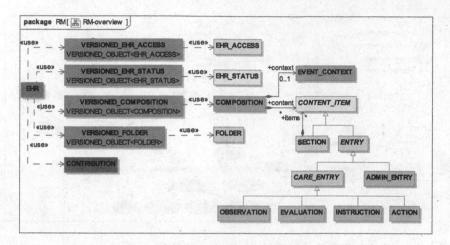

Fig. 2. EHR information model overview

define the semantics of all the 'hard' information in the record. The ENTRY package is divided as clinical and non-clinical information, i.e. the CARE_ENTRY and ADMIN_ENTRY classes, which is the generic structures for recording clinical statements. The former contains classes expressing information of any clinical activity in the care process around the patient, such as OBSERVATION is for all observed phenomena, including mechanically or manually measured, and responses in interview; EVALUATION is for assessments, diagnoses and plans; INSTRUCTION is for actionable statements such as medication orders, recalls, monitoring, reviews; and ACTION is for information recorded as a result of performing Instructions. The ADMIN_ENTRY class is used to capture administrative information.

4.3   The Personal Health Record Ontology Model

Either the HL7 V3 RIM or the openEHR IM is considered for organizing the health-related information on an individual that can be created, managed, and consulted by authorized clinicians and staff across more than one healthcare organization, which conforms to nationally recognized interoperability standards. However, a PHR is mainly focus on *personal* and is those parts of the EHR that an individual person could own and control. Based on the ENTRY concept in the openEHR IM and considering the six back-bone classes in the HL7 V3 RIM, we develop the PHR ontology model, as shown in Fig. 3, to illustrate the generic concepts and its relationships in PHRs, in which both observation-based and intervention-based information, and their dimension-related features are concerned.

In order to communicate with other EHR systems, the PHR ontology model has the similar structure to the Clinical Investigator Recording (CIR) ontology [27], which also accepted in the openEHR IM. Therefore, the PHR ontology model presented in this paper is well interoperable with other health systems.

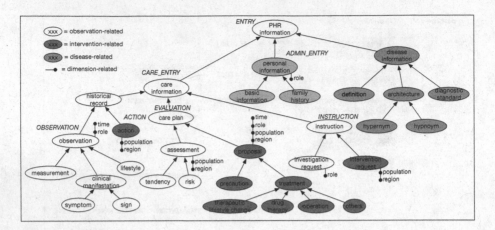

Fig. 3. The Personal Health Record (PHR) ontology model

The top-level categories in the ontology model are `care information`, `personal information` and `disease information`. The `care information` category encompasses all information that might be recorded at any point during the PHR management process, and consists of the major subcategories `historical record`, `care plan` and `instruction`. The `personal information` covers information on individuals, including `demographics`, such as *dob, sex, height, weight, pregnancy*, etc., and `family history`, such as *genetic genes, susceptible diseases*, etc., which is a type of administrative information with the role dimension feature. The `disease information` describes the definition, architecture, and diagnostic criteria of the diseases.

The `historical record` class corresponds to measurement and practise series which occur during the individual's daily life. The instances of `observation` class record the observation of any phenomenon or state of interest to do with the individual, including blood pressure readings, exercise levels, diet amounts, daily dosage, and so on, while the instances of `action` class are intervention activities according to the `care plan` and `instruction` events that have population and region dimension features.

In addition to the `measurement` subclass recording blood pressure and weight, which is associated with the monitoring and management of chronic diseases, `observation` has the subcategories `lifestyle` and `clinical manifestation`. The `lifestyle` class records exercise, smoking/tobacco, alcohol, drug use information and so on, which all have time and role dimension features, and the instances of `clinical manifestation` class record personal symptom and sign information. The `care plan` contains subclasses `assessment` and `proposal`, which are used to describe the evaluation statements and suggestions for personal health. The `tendency` and `risk` assessments have population and region dimensional features, i.e. different people and area have different evaluation criteria, and the `precaution` and `treatment` proposals have population, region, role and time dimensional features.

The `instruction` is used to specify the observation and action requests according to the requirements of medical workers, which enables simple and complex specifications to be expressed, including `investigation request` and `intervention request`. The role, population and region dimension features are considered in the `instruction` class respectively.

The PHR ontology model presented in this paper takes existing health record standards into account, i.e. HL7 V3 and openEHR, it has more advantages over individual health records in terms of managing personal health data. Furthermore, the PHR ontology model also incorporates a category of "disease", which is beneficial to understanding the disease concept when using PHR to manage individual health. Data in personal health archives has multidimensional characteristics, such as discussion, time, region and population characteristics. By describing the multidimensional features of these data, the occurrence, development, prevention and treatment of disease can be well documented. Categories represented in the ontology model are enabled by using prototype designing to express the information of interest in a PHR management system. We would note that even if the ontology model shown in this paper is not complete, the prototype might be constructed to account for each improved idea of what such categories should really be.

4.4   The Hypertension PHR Ontology Model

The establishment of a complete PHR ontology model requires two aspects: the basic framework of the PHR ontology model and data elements needed to be managed by the PHR. In the construction of specific disease domain model, data elements related to disease etiologies, pathogenesis, clinical manifestations, diagnosis and treatment methods, need to be defined and added into the underlying PHR basic framework. In this way, this article constructs a hypertension PHR ontology model.

Compared to the basic framework of PHR ontology model, the hypertension PHR ontology model contains more complete and specific contents of disease, personal, medical and health services information. For example, the `diagnostic standard` in the `disease information` records resting blood pressure values of upper arm brachial arteries, which can be used for hypertension diagnoses. In the `family history` part, more than 30 genetic information in chromosomal segments possibly related to hypertension are recorded.

In the `care information` section, this kind of materialization is more obvious. In the `lifestyle` part, information of daily potassium/sodium intakes and average daily exercise durations would be recorded, while in the `measurement` part, the records include projects of blood potassium, fasting blood glucose, total cholesterol, echocardiography, various plasma renin activities and other inspection items related to hypertension. In the `clinical manifestation` part, information of headache, dizziness and other symptoms, vascular murmur, heart murmur and other signs are recorded in details. The `tendency` records hypertension grades, the `risk` records important factors affecting hypertension prognoses of patients, and the `treatment` might even contain dose and medication times of five kinds of antihypertensive drugs.

In general, according to the constructed hypertension PHR ontology model, each information related to the occurrence and development of hypertension would be documented.

5 Conclusion and Future Work

This paper analyzes the multidimensional feature of Personal Health Records, and based on the HL7 V3 RIM and openEHR IM, we propose an ontology model of PHRs which is a high-level description of the PHR concepts and concerning multidimensional modelling for the PHR management. In addition, based on the PHR ontology model, we established a specific disease domain model—hypertension PHR ontology model. This is the foundation of establishing a PHR management system which takes multidimensional features of PHR into account. In this kind of PHR management system, personal health-related information can be well organized and shown, which is conducive to vigilance on individuals health status and beneficial for hospital, health care institutions, insurance companies to take appropriate health care measures to ensure personal health. Generally, our contributions can be further used in terms the following purposes, which also indicates our future work:

(1) Establishing a complete PHR ontology model that contains information about the occurrence and development of various diseases, and validating the PHR ontology model whit the aid of domain experts;
(2) Defining information interested in a PHR management system, including personal data collected by health monitoring devices, care plans for individual health living requests, health knowledge and assessment criteria for healthcare activities, and interoperation standards between different healthcare systems;
(3) Modelling processes of collecting PHR data, performing observation activities, generating care plans and concluding health reports for individuals, which compose the essential workflows in a PHR management system;
(4) Designing prototype of a PHR management system, including entity models, semantics specific to each information, processing workflows, deployment and integration architectures, user interfaces and interoperation standards;
(5) Implementing the PHR management system within a specific purpose along with the PHR ontology model.

Acknowledgement. This paper is supported by the Chinese NSFC International Cooperation and Exchange Program, *Research on Intelligent Home Care Platform based on Chronic Diseases Knowledge Management* (71661167007), and the Foundation of Key Research Institute of Humanities and Social Science at Universities, Chinese MoE (16JJD870002).

References

1. Emr vs ehr vs phr (2016). http://ed-informatics.org/healthcare_it_in_a_nutshell_2/emr_vs_ehr_vs_phr/
2. Hl7 reference information model (2016). http://www.hl7.org/implement/standards/rim.cfm
3. openehr architecture overview (2016). http://www.openehr.org/releases/BASE/latest/docs/architecture_overview/architecture_overview.html
4. Karshenas, S., Niknam, M.: Ontology-based building information modeling. In: Computing in Civil Engineering, pp. 476–483 (2013)
5. Yan, C.: Study on digital library knowledge organization based on ontology. Inf. Res. (9), 38–41 (2010)
6. Pandey, S.R., Panda, K.C.: Semantic solutions for the digital libraries based on semantic web technologies. Ann. Libr. Inf. Stud. (ALIS) **61**(4), 286–293 (2015)
7. Mi, Y., Cao, J.: A case study of semantic annotation with multi-ontology by upper-level ontology unitive controls. New Technol. Libr. Inf. Serv. (09), 36–41 (2012)
8. Shen, Z., Tang, Q., Fan, B.: Knowledge representation of an ontology for guidingan imaging reporting quality control knowledge base. China Digital Med. **10**(5), 89–91 (2015)
9. Ismail, S., Alshmari, M., et al.: A granular ontology model for maternal and child health information system. J. Healthcare Eng. (11), 1–9 (2017)
10. Casselman, R.M., Samson, D.: Moving beyond tacit and explicit: four dimensions of knowledge. In: Proceedings of the 38th Annual Hawaii International Conference on System Sciences (HICSS 2005), p. 243b (2005)
11. Goeken, M., Knackstedt, R.: Multidimensional reference models for data warehouse development. In: ICEIS 2007 - Proceedings of the Ninth International Conference on Enterprise Information Systems, Volume Eis, Funchal, Madeira, Portugal, June 2007
12. Guo, W., Zhang, X.: Description of ontology modules based on granularity. New Technol. Libr. Inf. Serv. **189**(2), 1–6 (2010)
13. Lv, Y., Zhao, G., Miao, P., Guan, Y.: Construction of multidimensional dynamic knowledge map based on knowledge requirements and knowledge connection. In: Wen, Z., Li, T. (eds.) Knowledge Engineering and Management. AISC, vol. 278, pp. 83–94. Springer, Heidelberg (2014). doi:10.1007/978-3-642-54930-4_9
14. Xu, X., Fang, D., Jiang, X.: Research on knowledge granularity representation and standardization during knowledge organization. Doc. Inf. Knowl. (6), 14 (2014)
15. Wang, F., Bi, Q.: Study on irregular knowledge lattice of multidimensional knowledge organization. Inf. Stud. Theory Appl. (01), 1–8 (2016)
16. Basic architecture and data standard of health record (2016). http://www.gov.cn/gzdt/2009-05/19/content_1319085.htm
17. Li, Q., Li, G.: Status and expectation of individual healthcare record r elated standards. Chongqin Med. **31**(21), 2398–2400 (2008)
18. Zhang, X., Yao, Z.: Modelling personal health record based on openehr. Comput. Appl. Softw. **30**(5), 71–73 (2013)
19. Xie, L., Yu, C., et al.: Personal health record based on XML. Comput. Appl. Softw. **27**(3), 152–155 (2010)
20. Huang, Y., Qian, Z. et al.: Building knowledge base for electronic health record based on ontology. China Digital Med. 06(4) (2011)
21. Tang, P., Ash, J., Bates, D., et al.: Personal health records: definitions, benefits, and strategies for overcoming barriers to adoption. J. Am. Med. Inf. Assoc. **13**(2), 121–126 (2006)

22. Roelofsen, Y., Hendriks, S.H., Sieverink, F., et al.: Differences between patients with type 2 diabetes mellitus interested and uninterested in the use of a patient platform (e-vitadm-2/zodiac-41). J. Diabetes Sci. Technol. **8**(2), 230–237 (2014)

23. Wagner, P.J., Dias, J., Howard, S., et al.: Personal health records and hypertension control: a randomized trial. J. Am. Med. Inf. Assoc. **19**(4), 626–634 (2012)

24. Schnipper, J.L., Gandhi, T.K., et al.: Effects of an online personal health record on medication accuracy and safety: a cluster-randomized trial. J. Am. Med. Inf. Assoc. **19**(5), 728–734 (2012)

25. Bahga, A., Madisetti, V.K.: A cloud-based approach for interoperable electronic health records (ehrs). IEEE J. Biomed. Health Inf. **17**(5), 894–906 (2013)

26. Zhang, J.: Study on personal health record service system under cloud environment. Chongqing Med. **44**(10), 1421–1423 (2015)

27. Beale, T., Heard, S.: An ontology-based model of clinical information. Stud. Health Technol. Inf. **129**(1), 760–4 (2007)

Constructing Knowledge Graphs of Depression

Zhisheng Huang[1(✉)], Jie Yang[2], Frank van Harmelen[1], and Qing Hu[1]

[1] Department of Computer Science, VU University Amsterdam,
Amsterdam, The Netherlands
{huang,Frank.van.Harmelen,qhu400}@cs.vu.nl
[2] Beijing Anding Hospital, Beijing, China
jieyangadyy@ccmu.edu.cn

Abstract. Knowledge Graphs have been shown to be useful tools for integrating multiple medical knowledge sources, and to support such tasks as medical decision making, literature retrieval, determining healthcare quality indicators, co-morbodity analysis and many others. A large number of medical knowledge sources have by now been converted to knowledge graphs, covering everything from drugs to trials and from vocabularies to gene-disease associations. Such knowledge graphs have typically been *generic*, covering very large areas of medicine. (e.g. all of internal medicine, or arbitrary drugs, arbitrary trials, etc.). This has had the effect that such knowledge graphs become prohibitively large, hampering both efficiency for machines and usability for people. In this paper we show how we use multiple large knowledge sources to construct a much smaller knowledge graph that is focussed on single disease (in our case major depression disorder). Such a disease-centric knowledge-graph makes it more convenient for doctors (in our case psychiatric doctors) to explore the relationship among various knowledge resources and to answer realistic clinical queries (This paper is an extended version of [1].).

1 Introduction

Major depressive disorder (MDD) has become a serious problem in modern society. It is an often-occurring disease for which no readily available treatment is available. It negatively affects a person's family, work or school life, and general health. Approximately 253 million people suffer from depression, about 3.6% of the global population (2013 figures). In the U.S., 1 in 10 Americans are affected by depression at one point in their life. Between 2–7% of adults with MDD die by suicide [2]. Using antidepressants has been considered the dominant treatment for MDD. However, between 30% to 50% of the individuals treated with antidepressants do not show a response. Hence, psychiatric doctors confront the challenge to make clinical decision efficiently by gaining a comprehensive analysis over various knowledge resources about depression.

In this paper we propose an approach to constructing a knowledge graph of depression using semantic web technology to integrate those knowledge resources. Semantic web technology allows us to achieve a high degree of interoperability over heterogeneous knowledge resources about depression. With a

© Springer International Publishing AG 2017
S. Siuly et al. (Eds.): HIS 2017, LNCS 10594, pp. 149–161, 2017.
https://doi.org/10.1007/978-3-319-69182-4_16

single semantic query over integrated data and knowledge resources, psychiatric doctors can be much more efficient in finding answers to queries which currently require to explore multiple databases about depression and make a time-consuming analysis on the results of searches.

The term "Knowledge Graph" is widely used to refer to a large scale semantic network consisting of entities and concepts as well as the semantic relationships among them, using representation languages such as RDF and RDF Schema [3]. Such knowledge graphs are used in the construction of many knowledge-based applications in medicine: extracting information from patient records [4], personalised medicine [5], support for co-morbidity analysis [6], data integration on drugs and their interactions [7], and many others.

Medical knowledge graphs typically cover very wide areas of medical knowledge: all proteines (UniProt), many known disease-gene associations (DisGeNet), as many drugs as possible (Drugbank), as many drug-drug interactions as are known (Sider), and massively integrated knowledge graphs such as Bio2RDF[1] and LinkedLifeData[2]. Such knowledge graphs are very *a-specific* in terms of the diseases that they cover, and are often prohibitively large, hampering both efficiency for machines and usability for people.

In this paper, we propose an approach to the construction of *disease-centric knowledge graphs*, which are specifically focussed on a single disease or coherent group of diseases. Our claims are (i) it is indeed possible to make disease-centric subgraphs without having to include the entire original graph, and (ii) that realistic clinical queries can still be answered over such disease-specific knowledge graphs without substantial loss of recall.

We illustrate our general idea by integrating various knowledge resources about depression (e.g., clinical trials, antidepressants, medical publications, clinical guidelines, etc.). We call the generated knowledge graph *DepressionKG* for short. The resulting set of integrated knowledge- and data-sources about depression is represented in RDF/NTriple format [3]. DepressionKG provides a data infrastructure to explore the relationship among various knowledge and data-sources about depression. We show how it provides support for clinical question answering and knowledge browsing.

2   Challenges

In order to integrate various knowledge resources of depression, we had to confront the following challenges:

– *Heterogeneity*. Different knowledge resources are generated by multiple creators. We have to achieve inter-operability among those knowledge resources. Beyond the ability of two or more computer systems to exchange information, semantic inter-operability is the ability to automatically interpret the

---

[1] http://bio2rdf.org/.
[2] http://linkedlifedata.com/.

exchanged information meaningfully and accurately in order to produce useful results as defined by the end users of both systems. To achieve semantic inter-operability, both sides must refer to a common information exchange reference model. The content of the information exchange requests are unambiguously defined, namely, what is sent is the same as what is understood.
– *Free text processing.* Often, some or all of the contents of our knowledge resources were not structured or even semi-structured, but instead contained a lot of free text. We have to use a natural language processing tool with a medical terminology to extract semantic relations from free text.
– *Partiality, inconsistency, and incorrectness.* Knowledge resources are not always complete. They usually contain some partial, inconsistent, or noisy (i.e., erroneous) data. We have to consider the partiality of those knowledge resources and develop efficient methods to deal with the partiality.
– *Expressive Representation* of Medical Knowledge. The formal language of Knowledge Graphs (up to OWL DL) is a decidable fragment of first order logic. Triples in knowledge graphs are expressed in even less expressive languages such as RDF and RDF Schema. Such languages are usually not expressive enough for medical knowledge representation.

In this paper we present some methods for dealing with the first two challenges while constructing a knowledge graph of depression, while leaving the third and fourth challenges for future work. We will show how DepressionKG can be used in some realistic scenarios for clinical decision support. We have implemented a system of DepressionKG aimed at psychiatric doctors with no background knowledge in knowledge graphs.

The rest of this paper is organized as follows. Section 3 presents the basics of knowledge graphs. Section 4 discusses various knowledge resources which can be used for making DepressionKG. Section 5 presents our methods to achieve the inter-operability and free text processing. Section 6 discusses several use cases of DepressionKG, and Sect. 7 reports our implementation of the DepressionKG system and the functionalities of the system. Section 8 discusses future work and conclusions.

3   Knowledge Graphs

Following commonly used technology, we will construct our knowledge graph as an RDF graph. Formally, an RDF graph is a collection of triples $\langle s, p, o \rangle$, each consisting of a subject s, a predicate p and an object o. Each triple represents a statement of a relationship p between the things denoted by the nodes s and o that it links. Identifiers for both p, s and o are URI's (Uniform Resource Identifier), allowing triples in one knowledge graph to refer to elements in another knowledge graph that resides in a physically different location. Besides a URI, the object o of a triple $\langle s, p, o \rangle$ can also be a literal (roughly: a string or any other XML-sanctioned datatype). Whereas objects that are denoted by URI's can themselves be the subject of other triples (giving rise to the graph construction), literals cannot be themselves the subject of other triples. Summarising, let U be the set of all URI, and L be the set of all literals. A knowledge graph K can be defined as a set of three-place tuples $\langle s, p, o \rangle$, with $s, p \in U$ and $o \in U \cup L$.

The languages RDF and RDF Schema [3] assign a fixed semantics to some of the predicates p. Examples of these are the predicates `rdf:type` to denote membership of a type, `rdfs:subClassOf` to denote (transitive) containment of subclasses, `rdfs:domain` and `rdfs:range` to denote membership of any subject resp. object of a given predicate to a specified type. These (and other) predefined predicates allow for automatic inference of additional triples from a given knowledge graph.

As a simple example, we state the basic properties of a clinical trial:

```
ct:NCT01178255 rdf:type ct:ClinicalTrial.
ct:NCT01178255 ct:ID"NCT01178255".
ct:NCT01178255 ct:BriefTitle
   "Efficacy and Safety of Homeopathy for Moderate Depression".
```

This example shows the use of name space abbreviations, writing `rdf:type` instead of http://www.w3.org/1999/02/22-rdf-syntax-ns#type

These triples state that that `ct:NCT01178255` is an instance of the concept `ClinicalTrial` with the given name (second triple) and title (third triple).

4   Knowledge Resources

In the present version of DepressionKG, we focus on knowledge resources relevant to the use of antidepressants. With this focus in mind, we have collected the following knowledge resources:

- *PubMed.* We used the keyword "depression" to search for publications in PubMed[3] from the semantic data set of Linked Life Data and obtained 46,060 publications. This search also includes results by using stemming keywords such as "depressive". This PubMed data set contains the basic data of a publication: authors, title of paper, journal name, publication date, abstract of the paper, PubMed ID (PMID), DOI, and its MeSH Terms.
- *Clinical Trials.* We searched for clinical trials on depression on ClinicalTrials.gov[4] and downloaded 10,190 studies (till January 23, 2017) with all study and result fields as XML data. We then converted those XML data into RDF triples. The basic data of clinical trials includes Trial ID, title of trial, agency, authority, brief summary, detailed description, completion status, starting date, study type and design, phase, eligibility criteria, reference, MeSH terms.
- *Medical Guidelines.* We have obtained several medical guidelines of depression such as the American guidelines for Major depression disorder, the NICE guideline for depression and others. So far we have converted only the text

---

[3] https://www.ncbi.nlm.nih.gov/pubmed/?term=depression.
[4] https://clinicaltrials.gov.

of the American depression guideline for primary care (2013) into the semantic representation we have designed for evidence-based medical guidelines [8]. The basic data about an evidence-based guideline includes title, publication year, version, topics, conclusion evidence class, and its evidences (as PubMed IDs).

– *DrugBank.* The DrugBank database[5] is a bioinformatics and cheminformatics resource that combines detailed drug data with comprehensive drug target (i.e. sequence, structure, and pathway) information. The current version of the database contains 4770 drug entries.

– *Wikipedia Antidepressant.* We obtained various webpages from Wikipedia about antidepressants and converted the basic data at those pages into a set of RDF Triples. DBPedia (dbpedia.org/), the RDF representation of facts from Wikipedia, was not sufficiently semantically rich for our use-case.

– *DrugBook.* We obtained various online manual and instruction books on antidepressants and converted key information into RDF Triples. So far, we have collected data of 264 antidepressants, covering the English and Chinese name of an antidepressant, ingredients, indications, side effects, caution, usage, pharmacological and toxicological data, producer, etc.

– *SIDER.* SIDER contains information on marketed drugs and their recorded adverse drug reactions[6]. The available information includes side effect frequency, drug and side effect classifications as well as links to further information, for example drugtarget relations.

– *UMLS.* The Unified Medical Language System (UMLS) integrates key terminology, classification and coding standards. UMLS covers well known medical terminologies such as MeSH, LOINC, SNOMED CT, and the UMLS concept hierarchy.

The current version of DepressionKG (version 0.60) consists of the RDF representation of the above knowledge resources. In addition, we add the data on MDD patients, which is generated by using APDG, a knowledge-based realistic patient data generator [9]. This allowed us to explore knowledge with respect to a specific patient for the demonstration of the DepressionKG system. A summary of DepressionKG is shown in Table 1. This shows that the resulting knowledge graph is only of moderate size (8.9M triples), whereas many of the original knowledge graphs are many times larger than this (10M-100M triples). In Sect. 6 we will illustrate that we can still answer a diversity of clinically relevant questions with such a small disease-centric knowledge graph.

Our 8.9M triples are dominated by the size of SNOMED CT. We decided to include all of SNOMED CT (instead of only those parts of the hierarchies relevant to depression) because some of the clinical use-cases presented to us by our psychiatric experts concern co-morbidities (eg. Alzheimer disease is a frequent co-morbidity with MDD), and overly restricting SNOMED CT would have hampered such co-morbidity queries.

---

[5] https://www.drugbank.ca/.
[6] http://sideeffects.embl.de/.

Table 1. DepressionKG version 0.6

Knowledge resource	Number of data item	Number of triple
ClinicalTrial	10,190 trials	1,606,446
PubMed on depression	46,060 papers	1,059,398
Medical guidelines	1 guideline	1,830
DrugBank	4,770 drugs	766,920
DrugBook	264 antidepressants	13,046
Wikipedia antidepressant side effects	17 antidepressants	6,608
SIDER	1,169 drugs	193,249
SNOMED CT		5,045,225
Patient data	1,000 patients	200,000
Total		**8,892,722**

5   Integration

We use the following four methods to integrate the various knowledge resources.

- *Direct Entity identification.* Some knowledge resources refer to the same entity with identical names, e.g. the PubMed IDs used in both PubMed and the clinical trials. Such identical entities are obvious links between these knowledge sources.
- *Direct Concept identification.* Numerous knowledge resources can be integrated by using direct *concept* identification. For example, both a publication in PubMed and a clinical trial are annotated with MeSH terms. This provides us with a way to detect a relationship between a clinical trial and a publication directly.
- *Semantic Annotation with an NLP tool.* We used Xerox's NLP tool XMedlan [10,11] for semantically annotating medical text (both concept identification and relation extraction) with medical terminologies such as SNOMED CT. We use XMedLan rather than similar terminology-based concept identifiers, such as the MetaMap system [12] or the BioPortal text annotator[7], because it is easier to adapt. XMedlan can be customized using a single command line with any subset from UMLS-integrated terminologies and even with in-house, non-standard terminologies [10].
- *Semantic Queries with regular expressions.* The previous three approaches are offline approaches to integrate knowledge sources. Semantic Queries with regular expressions are an online approach, because such queries find relationships among knowledge resources at query time. Although online method lead to more latency when getting query results, they do provide a method to detect a connection among different knowledge resources based on free text.

---

[7] https://bioportal.bioontology.org/annotator.

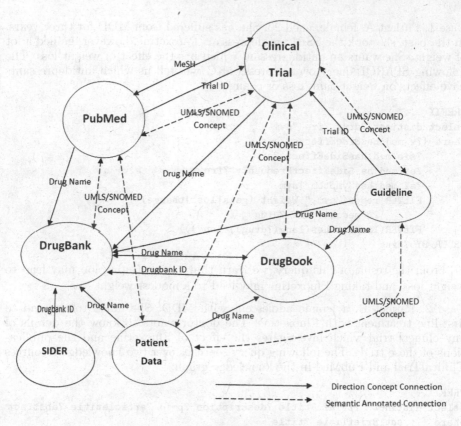

Fig. 1. Connectionality of DepressionKG

Figure 1 shows the connectivity of DepressionKG via direct concept identification and semantic annotation with medical concepts. An arrow denotes a direct concept connection from one knowledge resource to another via a property, and a dashed arrow denotes a semantic annotation connection via a concept identification in a medical terminology by using an NLP tool. The figure shows that our set of knowledge resources is well integrated.

6   Use Cases

In this section, we will discuss several use cases how the knowledge graph on depression can be used by psychiatric doctors for clinical decision support through SPARQL queries over the knowledge graphs. Making those queries requires knowledge of semantic web standards and the structure of the knowledge graph, and we would not expect a doctor to formulate those queries. Instead, such queries can be designed by the system developers and then used as a template for a user to change the parameters in the template to make their own queries. Furthermore, the queries can be wrapped in a user-friendly GUI.

Case 1. Patient A, female, aged 20. She has suffered from MDD for three years. In the past, she took the SSRI antidepressant Paroxetine, however, gained a lot of weight. She wants an antidepressant which has the effect of weight loss. The following SPARQL query over depressionKG will tell us which antidepressants have effects on weight gain, loss or change:

```
PREFIX ...
select distinct ?drug ?fre ?sym
where {?w med:hasSideEffects ?sfs.
       ?sfs med:hasSideEffect ?sf.
       ?sf med:hasSideEffectFrequency ?fre.
       ?sf med:hasSymptom ?sym.
       FILTER regex(?sym,"^Weight (gain|loss|change)")
             ?w med:hasName ?drug.
       FILTER(langMatches(lang(?drug), "en"))}
ORDER BY ?drug
```

From the result of this query, we learn that taking Bupropion may lead to weight loss, and taking Fluoxetine may lead to a modest weight loss.

Case 2. Patient B, a female adolescent with MDD. She failed to respond to first-line treatment with Fluoxetine. The doctor wants to know the details of any clinical trial which investigates the effect of Fluoxetine and the publications of those trials. The following query searches over two knowledge resources ClinicalTrial and PubMed in the knowledge graph:

```
PREFIX ...
select distinct  ?trial ?title ?description ?pmid ?articletitle ?abstract
where {?t sct:BriefTitle ?title.
       FILTER regex(?title, "Fluoxetine")
       ?t sct:NCTID ?trial.
       ?t sct:DetailedDescription ?description.
       ?pmid pubmed:hasAbstractText ?abstract.
       FILTER regex(?abstract,?trial)
       ?pmid pubmed:hasArticleTitle ?articletitle.}
```

This query finds three relevant trials, one with two publications, the others with one publication.

Case 3. Patient C, an adult male, suffers from mood disorder and hopes to try a clinical trial on depression. His clinical doctor wants to find an on-going trial which uses a drug intervention with target "neurotransmitter transporter activity". This requires a search that covers both DrugBank and ClinicalTrial. From DrugBank we know which the drug target, and then from ClinicalTrial we can know which trial has an intervention with the required drugs:

```
PREFIX ...
select distinct ?title  ?startdate ?trial ?drug
where {?d drugbank:genericName ?drug.
       ?d drugbank:target ?t.
       ?t drugbank:goClassificationFunction
          "neurotransmitter transporter activity" .
```

```
?s sct:InterventionName ?drug.
?ct sct:Intervention ?s.
?ct sct:NCTID ?trial.
?ct sct:BriefTitle ?title.
?ct sct:StartDate ?startdate.}
```

This query returns 25 clinical trials whose starting date is in 2016, and which meet the specified condition.

Case 4. Patient D, male, aged 45, has complained a lot that the antidepressant Clomipramine has lead to fatigue. Indeed fatigue is a very common side effect of Clomipramine. The psychiatric doctor wants to know if there exists any other antidepression drug of the same class where fatigue is a rare or uncommon side effect:

```
PREFIX ...
select distinct ?drug
where {?sf med:hasSymptom "Fatigue".
       ?sf med:hasSideEffectFrequency ?fre.
       FILTER regex(?fre,"(rare|uncommon)")
       ?sfs med:hasSideEffect ?sf.
       ?d med:hasSideEffects ?sfs.
       ?d  med:hasName ?drug.
       FILTER(langMatches(lang(?drug), "en"))
       ?c rdfs:label ?drug.
       ?c2 skos:narrower ?c.
       ?c1 skos:broader ?c2.
       ?c1 rdfs:label "Clomipramine"@en.}
```

In this example, we use the predicate skos:narrower and skos:broader to search over the SNOMED concept hierarchy to find two sibling concepts (i.e. two antidepressants of the same class). The answer for this search is "Dosulepin". The predicates skos:narrower and skos:broader can be replaced with the predicate rdfs:subClassOf if we want to use the built-in reasoning.

All of these examples are realistic clinical queries which would require substantial time and effort for a psychiatric doctor to answer, having to combine information from multiple knowledge sources.

7   DepressionKG System

We have implemented the DepressionKG system with a graphical user interface, so that psychiatric doctors who are not familiar with semantic web technology can use the system to search for the knowledge they need and to explore the relationships among various knowledge resources about depression for clinical decision support. We use a similar architecture used in the SemanticCT system [13] to implement the DepressionKG system. The DepressionKG system is built on the top of the LarKC system, a platform for scalable semantic data processing [14]. The architecture of the DepressionKG system is shown in Fig. 2. DepressionKG Management plays a central role in the system. It launches a

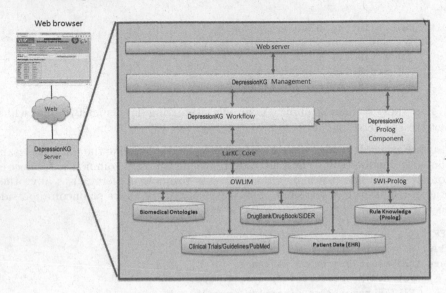

Fig. 2. Architecture of DepressionKG

web server which serves as the application interface of DepresionKG, so that the users can use a web browser to access the system locally (i.e., from the local-host) or remotely (i.e., via the Web). DepressionKG Management manages the SPARQL endpoints which are built as DepressionKG workflows. A generic reasoning plug-in in LarKC provides the basic reasoning service over semantic data of DepressionKG. The DepressionKG Management interacts with the DepressionKG Prolog component which provides the support for rule-based reasoning over the knowledge graph [15].

The DepressionKG system supports knowledge browsing and querying. A screenshot of the interface of the DepressionKG system is shown in Fig. 3. That screenshot also shows the result of a semantic query about the side-effects of antidepressants with respect to weight change. It will be deployed and evaluated in Beijing Anding Hospital, one of the biggest psychiatric hospitals in China, for experiments in the Smart Ward project, a case study in a Major International Cooperation Project between Beijing University of Technology (BJUT) and VU University Amsterdam, funded by the National Natural Science Foundation of China (2015-2019). The objective of the Smart Ward project is to develop a knowledge-based platform for monitoring and analyzing the status of patients and for supporting clinical decision making in a psychiatric ward. Therefore, we provided a bi-linguistic (English and Chinese) interface to the DepressionKG system. The deployment of the DepressionKG system in the Smart Ward project will be systematically evaluated in Beijing Anding Hospital, using realistic clinical scenarios from the hospital.

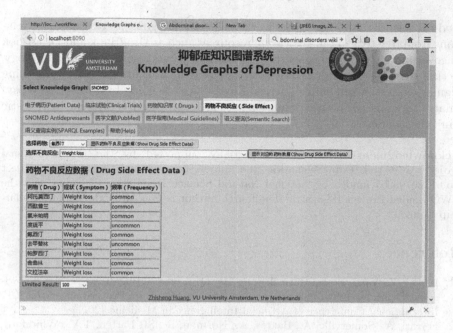

Fig. 3. Interface of the DepressionKG system

8 Discussion and Conclusion

Wide areas of related work can be used to improve our methods for knowledge graph selection and integration. Information extraction from freetext has been widely investigated. Various methods and tools can be used to construct knowledge graphs from large amount medical free text. In [4], Goodwin et al. propose an approach for automatic generation of a medical knowledge graph and show the usage of the knowledge graph for retrieving patient cohorts from electronic medical records. In [16], Paulheim provides a comprehensive survey of approaches and evaluation methods on knowledge graph refinement.

In this paper, we have proposed an approach to making a knowledge graph of depression, and we have shown how various knowledge resources concerning depression can be integrated for semantic inter-operability. We have provided several use cases for the knowledge graph of depression. From those use cases, we can see that by using a knowledge graph with its semantic search, it is rather convenient for the users to detect relationship which cover multiple knowledge resources. With the concept hierarchy of UMLS and its medical terminologies such as SNOMED CT, we can perform reasoning across the knowledge resources to gain a more comprehensive understanding on depression.

In future extensions of DepressionKG, we will add more knowledge resources which cover biomedical terminologies such as the Gene ontology GO, the protein ontology UNIPROT, ICD10, cell map, chemistry for life science, Human Phenotype Ontology, and others for the exploration from the perspective of basic medical sciences. Another future work is that we are going to extract more relations from free-text in the knowledge resources such as DrugBank and DrugBook to cover more structured properties, for example, indications and pharmacology, so that they can be integrated by direct concept identification, rather than using regular expressions in online queries. Finally, we are going to involve more psychiatric doctors to in the evaluation of the DepressionKG System in realistic clinical scenarios.

Acknowledgments. This work is partially supported by the Dutch national project COMMIT/Data2Semantics, the major international cooperation project No.61420106005 funded by National Natural Science Foundation of China, and the NWO-funded Project Re-Search. The fourth author is funded by the China Scholarship Council.

References

1. Huang, Z., Yang, J., van Harmelen, F., Hu, Q.: Constructing disease-centric knowledge graphs: a case study for depression (short version). In: Proceedings of the 2017 International Conference of Artificial Intelligence in Medicine (2017)
2. Ferrari, A., Somerville, A., Baxter, A., Norman, R., SB Patten, T.V., Whiteford, H.: Global variation in the prevalence and incidence of major depressive disorder: a systematic review of the epidemiological literature. Psychol. Med. **43**(3), 471–481 (2013)
3. Cyganiak, R., Wood, D., Lanthaler, M.: RDF 1.1 concepts and abstract syntax (2014)
4. Goodwin, T., Harabagi, S.M.: Automatic generation of a qualified medical knowledge graph and its usage for retrieving patient cohorts from electronic medical records. In: IEEE Seventh International Conference on Semantic Computing (2013)
5. Panahiazar, M., Taslimitehrani, V., Jadhav, A., Pathak, J.: Empowering personalized medicine with big data and semantic web technology: Promises, challenges, and use cases. In: IEEE International Conference on Big Data (2014)
6. Zamborlini, V., Hoekstra, R., Silveira, M.D., Pruski, C., ten Teije, A., van Harmelen, F.: Inferring recommendation interactions in clinical guidelines. Semantic Web **7**(4), 421–446 (2016)
7. Jovanovik, M., Trajanov, D.: Consolidating drug data on a global scale using linked data. J. Biomed. Semant. **8**(1), 3 (2017)
8. Huang, Z., ten Teije, A., van Harmelen, F., Ait-Mokhtar, S.: Semantic representation of evidence-based clinical guidelines. In: Proceedings of 6th International Workshop on Knowledge Representation for Health Care (KR4HC 2014) (2014)
9. Huang, Z., van Harmelen, F., ten Teije, A., Dentler, K.: Knowledge-based patient data generation. In: Riaño, D., Lenz, R., Miksch, S., Peleg, M., Reichert, M., ten Teije, A. (eds.) KR4HC/ProHealth -2013. LNCS, vol. 8268, pp. 83–96. Springer, Cham (2013). doi:10.1007/978-3-319-03916-9_7
10. Ait-Mokhtar, S., Bruijn, B.D., Hagege, C., Rupi, P.: Intermediary-stage ie components, D3.5. Technical report, EURECA Project (2014)
11. Khiari, A.: Identification of variants of compound terms, master thesis. Technical report, Universit Paul Sabatier, Toulouse (2015)
12. Aronson, A.R., Lang, F.: An overview of metamap: historical perspective and recent advances. J. Am. Med. Inform. Assoc.: JAMIA **17**(3), 229–236 (2010)

13. Huang, Z., ten Teije, A., van Harmelen, F.: SemanticCT: a semantically-enabled system for clinical trials. In: Riaño, D., Lenz, R., Miksch, S., Peleg, M., Reichert, M., ten Teije, A. (eds.) KR4HC/ProHealth -2013. LNCS, vol. 8268, pp. 11–25. Springer, Cham (2013). doi:10.1007/978-3-319-03916-9_2

14. Fensel, D., van Harmelen, F., Andersson, B., Brennan, P., Cunningham, H., Della Valle, E., Fischer, F., Huang, Z., Kiryakov, A., Lee, T., School, L., Tresp, V., Wesner, S., Witbrock, M., Zhong, N.: Towards LarKC: a platform for web-scale reasoning. In: Proceedings of the IEEE International Conference on Semantic Computing (ICSC 2008). IEEE Computer Society Press, CA (2008)

15. Huang, Z., den Teije, A., van Harmelen, F.: Rule-based formalization of eligibility criteria for clinical trials. In: Proceedings of the 14th Conference on Artificial Intelligence in Medicine (AIME 2013) (2013)

16. Paulheim, H.: Knowledge graph refinement: a survey of approaches and evaluation methods. Semantic Web 8(3), 489–508 (2017)

Constructing Three-Dimensional Models for Surgical Training Simulators

Marina Gavrilova[1], Stanislav Klimenko[2], Vladimir Pestrikov[2(✉)], and Arkadiy Chernetskiy[2]

[1] Department of Computer Science, University of Calgary, Calgary, Canada
[2] Institute of Computing for Physics and Technology,
Moscow Institute of Physics and Technology, Moscow, Russia
pestrikov@phystech.edu

Abstract. New technologies introduced into medicine necessitate training of medical personnel to operate new equipment and techniques. For this purpose, training simulators and educational materials should be provided to the medical staff involved. This work concerns creating 3D model of surgical field for simulators to promote minimally invasive surgery. The paper reports the modes of constructing a photorealistic model of surgical field from endoscopic video streams, SFM, SLAM methods, as well as the problem of surface reconstruction from a point cloud and texture mapping on the constructed model.

Keywords: Surgical training simulators · Minimal invasive surgery · Structure from motion · SFM · Simultaneous localization and mapping · SLAM · 3D reconstruction

1 Introduction

In the modern world, it is evident that the new technologies appear practically every day. Being popular and spreading widely the recent technology advances easily integrate in our lives, with no exception to the medicine. New technologies available in medicine necessitate the medical personnel to be properly trained to operate with the new equipment and to handle new techniques. Therefore, it is necessary to create training simulators and provide educational materials. This paper concerns with the creation of 3D model of the surgical field for training simulators, training minimally invasive surgery.

The minimally invasive surgery is highly beneficial compared to traditional open operations. The whole procedure assumes small instrumentally-made cuts. The main advantages imply low blood loss, lower traumatism, and rapid and less painful post-operational recovery period. But such low-invasive intervention requires special training for surgeons.

Surgeons need to adapt handling a camera and operating instruments, to become accustomed to their mutual arrangement while observing an operation on a special monitor. These are the reasons to create modern surgical training simulators. A crucial function of simulators is to provide detailed and plausible imaging of the surgical field.

© Springer International Publishing AG 2017
S. Siuly et al. (Eds.): HIS 2017, LNCS 10594, pp. 162–169, 2017.
https://doi.org/10.1007/978-3-319-69182-4_17

Thus, two major goals have to be reached: (1) to create qualitative and precise 3D model of surgical field, and (2) to map photorealistic textures on this model.

Firstly, the model should be properly constructed. There are two major approaches for constructing the operational field model: the construction may be done (1) by using the MRT data, medical atlases and other credible sources, the result of which can be exemplified by the ArthroS [1] simulator produced by EvenaMedical Company; or (2) by using photo- and video- images of real surgical operations, exemplified by scientific developments of A. Sourin [2–4].

In the second case, it is proposed to build a panoramic image of surgical field based on operation video. The relief model is then superposed on this panorama that a surgeon can interact with it and add three-dimensional models of target organs to the output. The drawbacks of this approach imply inaccuracy and distortions in transferring a voluminous object on a flat panorama, as well as a lack of possibility to utilize such model in simulator.

To avoid the above problems, it is suggested to begin with building of the 3D model of the surgical field using a video sequence. This procedure has got some advantages compared to constructing the model from the MRT data or biological atlases. It does not require preliminary location positioning, additional labels or an expensive preliminary examination (such as MRT or KT) as the implied method is based on information recovered from endoscopic images. In this case, the cost of creating each model is noticeably reduced. So, it is feasible to create the model of a particular object for its further detailed examination or for training and teaching purposes. For instance, a surgical field of appointed patient can be used as a source, the result of which might be helpful in modeling the course of a future operation. A surgeon can rehearse all complicated instances of a forthcoming operation, come across possible difficulties. In addition, it seems possible to create the models of particular clinical cases to be subsequently included into a scenario of personnel training.

For successful implementation, it is decided to use algorithms based on the Structure from Motion (SFM) and the Simultaneous Localization and Mapping (SLAM) methods. Noticeably, these methods, particularly SLAM, have been significantly developed recently.

The second part of this paper provides the basic steps of the SFM method. Then the paper introduces algorithms of the SLAM family. Further on, the modes of constructing 3D surfaces of the object and texture mapping onto the surface are described. The paper closes with the conclusion.

2 Principal Steps of SFM Method

The aim to construct 3D structures from a set of images (photographs or frames) taken from different perspectives is referred to as the structure from motion (SFM). It can be solved with the following procedure applied. At first, entry images should be analyzed to determine feature points. After that, coordinates of these points in three-dimensional space should be found using triangulation. In this respect the problem is to find the camera coordinates in the video source. With a sufficient amount of detected feature points in the images, it is possible to compare the number of equations to define both coordinates of cameras and of feature points.

Thus, the steps for solving the SFM problem have been formulated [5]:

- **Search for features on input images.** In most cases it is advised to apply either SIFT or SURF for solving the problem of searching and describing feature points. SIFT commonly detects more features on the image, but SURF is more quick and seems to be more robust.
- **Search for matches between the points found.** It is recommended to refer to FLANN with the big high-dimensional data sets. It is also advised to use linear methods establishing the best compliance for each point found with sparse data [6].
- **The false compliances filtration.** Preliminary selection may be done basing on the assumption of positioning of corresponding points as well as on heuristic methods. These points are further filtered by the RANSAC method [7].
- **The equation system processing, the estimation of camera position and the reconstruction of the 3D structure.**

3   Algorithms of SLAM Family

The method of Simultaneous Localization and Mapping (SLAM) is currently widely applied. The problem posed for the method is classic for robotics: in transferring the sensor in the unknown space over the unknown trajectory it is advised to construct 3D or flat map of the environment and locate a sensor. In the case, when this sensor presented with a video camera, the SLAM problem and the SFM problem looks similar in nature. In this case it is called visual-SLAM or VSLAM. One of the differences to distinguish in the SLAM method is real-time working with a video, rather than with a final set of photos. That is, not the entire set of images is handed over to the algorithm as an input. Instead, the input data are portioned.

Keeping in mind the aforementioned, the working time is critical for SLAM-based algorithms, and it is reasonable to use the video sequence in their application. The key differences between the video stream and photos in respect to the paper issue are minor camera shifts on the sequenced frames, as well as the possibility of tracing feature points. Besides, the algorithm data is applied for the positioning autonomous devices and systems, which it is difficult or impossible to supplement with big computing power. Therefore, one of the main requirements for SLAM family algorithms is the demand of low computing power.

Today, two major procedures for solving Visual SLAM problem are outlined:

- *Feature-based methods* – the methods based on searching for feature points on the image;
- *Direct methods* – direct methods analyzing an entire image.

Each method is presented with its significant algorithm with the *ORB-SLAM* algorithm stands as a sample for feature-based methods and the *LSD-SLAM* algorithm – for the direct ones.

3.1 ORB-SLAM

The basics of the ORB-SLAM [8] algorithm are very similar to those of SFM. However, such features of SLAM as real-time operating and constant data updating amend the algorithm. Tasks of updating and specifying the model (or map) of the environment, constructing and refinement of the camera route, searching for loops on the camera route and some others appear consequently. In order to be equal to these tasks ORB-SLAM is designed to use the ORB algorithm [9] for features search and description. The algorithm is proved to have extremely high working speed and gives out the results of acceptable quality.

The authors of ORB-SLAM proposed their method for the environment map initialization. Firstly, two frames that have a sufficient amount of coinciding features detected with the ORB detector are picked. Then, basing on the matches found it is necessary to locate the camera shift in respect to selected frames. For cases when the camera is moved slightly, or part of scene getting into a frame is flat, the camera shift should be calculated via homography. Otherwise, the camera shift is better described with a fundamental matrix. The main idea of the method is that the initial camera position is computed with the two models involved. Then they are compared in order to look for the best one. The initial map of environment is built with the selected model applied.

ORB-SLAM consists of three modules that operate in parallel streams:

- Tracking stands for the module responsible for locating the camera position on the current frame, as well as for making the decision to distinguish a current frame as the key frame;
- Local mapping stands for the module responsible for construction and refinement of the model (or map) of the environment from distinguished key points;
- Loop closing stands for the module that searches for closing loop of a camera if a new key frame appears; it also refines the camera tracking and environment map if the loop closing is discovered.

As a result of applying this algorithm, the camera route is described with the decent precision and the point's cloud of the geometry of the environment is generated. However, the algorithm may interrupt its work or provide wrong results in case when a part of the environment contains small amount of features.

3.2 LSD-SLAM

The main feature of the LSD-SLAM algorithm [10] is that it uses the entire image as information pool, in contrast to other algorithms, which are feature point-oriented. Below the main stages of this algorithm are considered.

LSD-SLAM includes three main modules namely the tracking module, module of depth map estimation and the module of environment map optimization:

- The tracking module is responsible for locating the camera on each new frame. The camera position is calculated relative to the current key frame position. The position of previous frame is used as the initial approximation.

- The depth map estimation attracts the processed frame for refinement or replacement of the current key frame. If the shift between the new frame and the current key frame is small enough, then the depth map of the current key frame is specified. Otherwise, the new frame becomes a key frame. The depth map of the previous key frame is taken as the initial approximation of the depth map for the new key frame.
- When a new key frame appears, the previous key frame, which is not to be changed further, is used for updating the environment map.

The original depth map of the first frame is initialized at random. In the meantime the environment map construction is suspended for some time, until the algorithm output is reliable enough.

The noticeable advantage of the second method is the independence of feature points that may be extremely useful while processing poorly textured objects often found on the videos of minimally invasive surgeries.

4   Reconstruction of Surface and Superposition of Textures

The result map of the SFM approach and some SLAM algorithms, e.g. ORB-SLAM, is presented as a points cloud. But in a general case the result cloud is insufficiently rare for constructing a photorealistic model of a good quality.

4.1   Construction of a Dense Points Cloud

The most popular solution of the problem of constructing a dense points cloud is the method proposed in the referenced article [11]. This method is available in the PMVS library [12]. Each point from the rare cloud is superposed by a *patch* that is a small oriented rectangular. The same is done with neighbor areas of the model. Then incorrectly superposed patches are filtered. The last two steps have several iterations before the patches cover the surface of the reconstructed model densely.

Each image the algorithm receives as an input is conventionally divided into similar sectors $C_i(x, y)$ in order approximate to the result in which every sector of each image contains the projection of at least one patch. The model of the patch p is described by the position of its center $c(p)$ and a unit normal vector $n(p)$.

A collection of images is picked for each patch showing the shared feature point. Some frames can be dismissed by the function of photometric error between the frames. Then parameters of a patch are specified via the minimization of photometric error between remaining frames. After that, when a corresponding patch is built for each point of the original points cloud, the algorithm comes over to the step of enlargement.

For each point of the image neighboring the cell that contains the patch p projection, the algorithm tries to build a new patch with the exception for the cells that already contains the projection of any patch. If the area of the model onto which a new patch p' is superposed has a significant height differences relatively to the area of the reference model containing the patch p, the attempt to impose this patch onto the image reveals an easily noticeable error. In such cases the patch p' is set as an overshoot and is discarded from the model. If the patch undergoes the described test, its parameters are specified via minimization of photometric error between the frames that contains the projection of this patch. After that, new patches are additionally filtered, and the process of constructing new patches is launched anew. The authors of the algorithm suggest repeating this procedure for at least three times.

Thus, in the algorithm output we get a new dense points cloud, after that it is possible to superpose meshes onto a scene and obtain the required surface.

4.2   Reconstruction of Model Surface from a Dense Points Cloud

After obtaining a dense points cloud, the surface model construction becomes accessible. This matter evolves a number of approaches, yet the authors of this paper consider the popular method of Poisson Surface Reconstruction [13] that available in the PMVS library most suitable.

The essence of this approach based on the observation that the vector field of internal normal of the solid body boundary may be interpreted as the membership function gradient of this body. The vector array may be taken as the vector field of the boundary. These vectors are inversed to patch normal obtained from the constructing of a dense cloud. Thus, the vector field $\vec{V} : R^3 \to R^3$ is obtained. It is necessary to find the scalar function $\chi : R^3 \to R^{\wedge}3$ minimizing the error function:

$$\chi = \int \left\| \nabla \chi(p) - \vec{V}(p) \right\|^2 dp \tag{1}$$

This problem is solving with the Poisson equation:

$$\Delta \chi = \nabla \cdot \vec{V} \tag{2}$$

Then the isosurface with a zero value of the function χ is found. The positive values of the function correspond to the original field of the model, while the negative ones - to external. All approaches and modifications improving the model are reported in the original paper.

4.3   Photorealistic Texture Mapping onto the Constructed Surface

Further on, it is necessary to map the textures onto the constructed 3D model. For this purpose the image of the due part of the model is projected on the surface of the constructed model from the positioned camera. The target part of the model is often found on more than one frame. So, it is critical to pick up the most appropriate frame for texture mapping. The following procedure is proposed for this particular instance. The points are estimated using several factors for each small part of 3D model. The list of these factors contains: (a) the distance from the model surface to the frame plane, (b) the angle between the frame and the surface normal, (c) the distance from the frame boundary (it is reasonable to map textures from the central part of a frame as optic distortions may occur on the periphery), (d) image definition, and (e) brightness (areas that over lit or too dark are fined). Finally each part of the model is filled in with a texture from the frame with the highest score.

In this case, however, one more issue might be the case. Due to the difference in lighting, minor inaccuracies in the model construction and some misinterpretation of the camera location, the boundaries of the image textures stitching could be quite distinguishable. Thus, it is essential to level out the brightness of different frames and smooth out the transitions using the Multi-band Blending [14].

In this research, the texture mapping is an important issue to consider. The above-proposed algorithm combined with the correct choice of the 3D model reconstruction techniques, result in building the top-quality realistic model of surgery field that is the principal goal of this work.

5   Conclusion

The paper reports various approaches to constructing 3D model of environment from the video sequence or the collection of separate pictures. Application of such algorithms facilitates the creation of the surgical field model applied in surgical training simulators, and requires no specialist involvement. It stimulates building diverse models for medical personnel training, operative intervention planning or diagnostics.

Using the SFM procedure it is feasible to get a photorealistic 3D model of the environment, but in terms of the goal posed this approach has some disadvantages. For instance, this algorithm operates with a final set of static photos, rather than with a video stream. This means that before launching the algorithm it is necessary to distinguish an appropriate set of frames from a video sequence, and only after that one can proceeds with the 3D model construction. The set of random frames of a video sequence as well as the choice of frames with set intervals may be far from meeting the requirements. Besides, such procedure cannot operate in real time and build the model concurrently with the shooting. On the other hand, the presence of the entire set of entry data allows a coherent model to be built at once.

The paper reports the other approach, involving the SLAM application. It mitigates the issues of the SFM method described above, as they operate with a video stream in real time. With such procedure, the necessary key frames are selected automatically by the program, providing more optimal data set to build the 3D model with. An important advantage of this family of algorithms is their ability to work in real time with relatively low computing power. Thus, it can be concluded that SLAM is more suitable for solving the assigned problem.

The article reports two major approaches to copying with SLAM issues: (1) the method based on searching for feature points and (2) the direct method of analyzing the entire image. Comparing these approaches, the benefits of the feature points-based methods are: high-speed operation overshoots handling, essential stability and initialization easiness. The basic benefits of direct methods are: the ability of the algorithms to operate with poorly textured objects as well as with a few feature points on the images; the building of a more dense stage model, in contrast to the sparse points cloud of the aforesaid methods; applying the big piece of information obtained from the image.

Working with different objects under varying conditions, either approach should be preferred.

References

1. Stunt, J.J., Kerkhoffs, G.M.M.J., van Dijk, C.N., Tuijthof, G.J.M.: Validation of the ArthroS virtual reality simulator for arthroscopic skills. Knee Surgery Sports Traumatol. Arthroscopy **23**(11), 3436–3442 (2014). doi:10.1007/s00167-014-3101-7

2. Rasool, S., Sourin, A., Pestrikov, V., Kagda, F.: Modeling arthroscopic camera with haptic devices in image-based virtual environments. In: 2014 IEEE Haptics Symposium (HAPTICS), pp. 403–408. IEEE (2014). doi:10.1109/haptics.2014.6775489

3. Pestrikov, V., Sourin, A.: Towards making panoramic images in virtual arthroscopy. In: 2013 International Conference on Cyberworlds, pp. 48–51. IEEE (2013). doi:10.1109/cw.2013.29

4. Rasool, S., Sourin, A.: Image-driven virtual simulation of arthroscopy. Vis. Comput. **29**(5), 333–344 (2012). doi:10.1007/s00371-012-0736-6

5. Hartley, R., Zisserman, A.: Multiple View Geometry in Computer Vision. Cambridge University Press, New York (2003). doi:10.1017/cbo9780511811685

6. Muja, M., Lowe, D.G.: Fast approximate nearest neighbors with automatic algorithm configuration. In: VISAPP 2009, pp. 331–340 (2009). doi:10.5220/0001787803310340

7. Fischler, M.A., Bolles, R.C.: Random sample consensus: a paradigm for model fitting with applications to image analysis and automated cartography. Commun. ACM **24**(6), 381–395 (1981). doi:10.1145/358669.358692

8. Mur-Artal, R., Montiel, J.M.M., Tardos, J.D.: ORB-SLAM: a versatile and accurate monocular SLAM system. IEEE Trans. Robot. **31**(5), 1147–1163 (2015). doi:10.1109/tro.2015.2463671

9. Rublee, E., Rabaud, V., Konolige, K., Bradski, G.: ORB: an efficient alternative to SIFT or SURF. In: 2011 International Conference on Computer Vision, pp. 2564–2571. IEEE (2011). doi:10.1109/iccv.2011.6126544

10. Engel, J., Schöps, T., Cremers, D.: LSD-SLAM: large-scale direct monocular SLAM. In: Fleet, D., Pajdla, T., Schiele, B., Tuytelaars, T. (eds.) ECCV 2014. LNCS, vol. 8690, pp. 834–849. Springer, Cham (2014). doi:10.1007/978-3-319-10605-2_54

11. Furukawa, Y., Ponce, J.: Accurate, dense, and robust multiview stereopsis. IEEE Trans. Pattern Anal. Mach. Intell. **32**(8), 1362–1376 (2010). doi:10.1109/tpami.2009.161

12. Furukawa, Y., Ponce, J.: Patch-based multi-view stereo software. http://www.di.ens.fr/pmvs. Accessed 10 June 2017

13. Kazhdan, M., Bolitho, M., Hoppe, H.: Poisson surface reconstruction. In: Symposium on Geometry Processing, pp. 61–70 (2006)

14. Burt, P.J., Adelson, E.H.: A multiresolution spline with application to image mosaics. ACM Trans. Graph. **2**(4), 217–236 (1983). doi:10.1145/245.247

A Framework for Automated Knowledge Graph Construction Towards Traditional Chinese Medicine

Heng Weng[1], Ziqing Liu[2], Shixing Yan[3], Meiyu Fan[1], Aihua Ou[1],
Dacan Chen[1(✉)], and Tianyong Hao[4(✉)]

[1] The Second Affiliated Hospital of Guangzhou University of Chinese Medicine,
Guangzhou, China
ww128@qq.com, 1175383819@qq.com, 4910702@163.com
[2] The Second Clinical Medical College, Guangzhou University of Chinese Medicine,
Guangzhou, China
lzq_lby@163.com
[3] Department of Control Science and Engineering, Tongji University, Shanghai, China
yanshixing@jindengtai.cn
[4] School of Information Science and Technology,
Guangdong University of Foreign Studies, Guangzhou, China
haoty@gdufs.edu.cn

Abstract. Medical knowledge graph can potentially help knowledge discovery from clinical data, assisting clinical decision making and personalized treatment recommendation. This paper proposes a framework for automated medical knowledge graph construction based on semantic analysis. The framework consists of a number of modules including a medical ontology constructor, a knowledge element generator, a structured knowledge dataset generator, and a graph model constructor. We also present the implementation and application of the constructed knowledge graph with the framework for personalized treatment recommendation. Our experiment dataset contains 886 patient records with hypertension. The result shows that the application of the constructed knowledge graph achieves dramatic accuracy improvements, demonstrating the effectiveness of the framework in automated medical knowledge graph construction and application.

Keywords: Knowledge graph · Semantic analysis · Personalized medical service

1 Introduction

With the fast prevalence and development of precision medicine, more and more patients are seeking personalized medical treatment services. This requires clinicians to continuously pay attention to the rapid development of medical research, and accumulate effective clinical treatment cases based on a large amount of domain knowledge. Clinicians also need to analyze and summarize historical treatment cases time by time. This bring a huge burden on clinicians of new knowledge learning from large amount of medical data in such an information exploration era [1].

© Springer International Publishing AG 2017
S. Siuly et al. (Eds.): HIS 2017, LNCS 10594, pp. 170–181, 2017.
https://doi.org/10.1007/978-3-319-69182-4_18

Medical data has the nature characteristics of big data including volume, variety, velocity, and veracity [2, 3], thus bringing challenges for the storing, transferring, and processing of continuously emerging medical data [4]. On the other hand, the developing data processing techniques provide opportunities for leveraging medical data to assist clinicians in many applications [5], e.g., medical decision support [6–8], medical knowledge mining [9, 10], drug discovery analytics [11, 12], etc. Therefore, considering the limited time of clinicians, extracting knowledge from medical data for personalized treatment are both necessary to assist clinicians and help them improve working efficiency.

Knowledge discovery based on Human-Computer Interaction (HCI) may be a promising approach for such purpose, as addressed by Holzinger [13]. In the knowledge discovery models, Knowledge Graph (KG) obtains increasingly attention in medical domain evidenced by its capability of predicting the cancer clinical treatment via the combination with other patient information such as gene [14]. Moreover, it has been successfully applied on the hyperosmolar byperglycemic state management for ICU adult patients [15]. KG can assist clinicians in retrieval and understanding the clinical practice guidelines and protocols as well. Consequently, KG can be used not only for mining potential hidden knowledge, but also for assisting clinicians in their academic research, clinical decision support, knowledge retrieval, etc.

To assist clinicians in high efficient knowledge learning and retrieval, this paper proposes a framework for Traditional Chinese Medicine (TCM) knowledge graph construction through the information extraction from existing clinical texts. The framework is based on a semantic analysis network containing a large amount of meta knowledge, as the nodes in the network. The constructed knowledge graph can be aggregated into structured vector representations according to different dimensions for the convenience of semantic distance calculation and semantic inference. According to the evaluation of medical dataset containing 866 real patient cases with hypertension, the result shows that the classification performance has been significantly improved by applying the constructed TCM knowledge graph. The experiments indicate that the proposed framework can help data modeling in knowledge graph construction, demonstrating its effectiveness. We also present how the constructed TCM knowledge graph can potentially benefit clinical application such as personalized treatment recommendation.

2   Related Work

Knowledge graph is a symbolic expression of the physical world, which generalizes the world into a logical link among all conceptual entities and attributes. From the perspective of the graph theory, knowledge graph is essentially a conceptual network in which the nodes represent the entities (or concepts) of the physical world, and the edges represent various semantic relations among the entities. The medical concepts are commonly organized in hierarchical structures while the relations among conceptual entities and attributes are intricate.

In Traditional Chinese Medicine (TCM) domain, there are some existing research works on TCM knowledge graph construction. Zhang et al. [16] addressed that the basic structure of TCM knowledge graph consisted of concept hierarchical relations and entity relations. They defined semantic inferences between the nodes according to general TCM knowledge. They regarded knowledge graph as a mapping between the relational tree of concepts and the relational graph of entities. However, the research only provided the application direction of TCM knowledge graph without offering practical application cases. Moreover, the semantic references still relied on the manual work of domain experts.

Yu et al. [17] focused on the concept organization of TCM and integrated the structured knowledge resource into a large-scale knowledge graph, which embedded with literature search, knowledge retrieval and other functions to provide knowledge navigation, integration and visualization services, etc. Based on an ontology, the knowledge graph was further divided into concept semantic network and thesaurus. The former defined the correlation among TCM concepts and knowledge resources, while the latter structured concepts and terms. The research reported some promising applications in KG visualization and ontology retrieval. However, the method still needed tedious manual work on semantic inference definition.

Shi et al. [18] claimed that a computation framework for Textual Medical Knowledge (TMK) is necessary to construct a TCM knowledge graph. They emphasized that the usage of framework needed to meet three requirements: (1) able to organize heterogeneous TMK and integrate with HIS data to transfer data; (2) should have reasonable knowledge element expressions supporting both human and machine interpretation to realize efficient retrieval; (3) should have a retrieval function to facilitate the promotion of latest knowledge to users. They constructed a healthcare organization model that contained three parts: Medical Knowledge Model (MKM), Health Data Model (HDM), and Terminology Glossary (TG), for organizing TMK into concept maps to define normalize Electronic Health Records (EHRs) and to provide the meta-thesaurus of TMK and HDM cases. It applied First-order Predicate Logic for semantic inference and adopted text categorization algorithms to rectified semantic inference errors. Yet, the application still has limitations on practical applications such as clinical prescription patterns summarization.

The existing works focused on the content-aware natural language processing. It was feasible for acquiring knowledge with explicit description. However, they seldom deal with hidden knowledge with implicit descriptions in medical texts, e.g., main syndrome and concurrent syndrome, prescription based on syndrome differentiation, etc. To that end, we propose a new automated extraction method for TCM knowledge graph construction. The purpose of the TCM knowledge graph is to realize automatic extraction of semantic inference, discovering hidden knowledge in accumulated treatment cases of experienced physicians and finding diagnose, treatment and prescription patterns, etc. The knowledge graph includes two kinds of the visualization of complex knowledge element associations. This research also applies deep learning technology to annotate each knowledge unit with individual coordinate mapping and distance information to express the correlation among knowledge elements, which can not only be used in data description of current TMK to bring clinic physicians convenience in understanding general ideas of data set, but also be applied in relevant research work such as couplet medicine retrieval, core prescription, single substance drug, etc.

3   The Framework

A knowledge graph construction framework based on the ontology model and deep learning technique is proposed. The framework aims to automate the meta knowledge extraction and conversion processes which transfer meta knowledge to vector representation for semantic distance calculation and semantic inference. The vector representation is used to regenerate structured datasets according to clinical scenario differences. The generated datasets can be stored into meta knowledge warehouse for further usage. Each sample of the dataset exists in a sparse matrix and is assigned with a list of labels, where the labels correspond to meta knowledge. The generated datasets are further used to train a Recurrent Neural Network (RNN) [19] model for calculating the semantic distance and relation paths of given meta knowledge to discover the potential hidden knowledge so as to construct a domain-specific knowledge graph. As shown in Fig. 1, the whole framework consist of four main modules including: (1) a medical

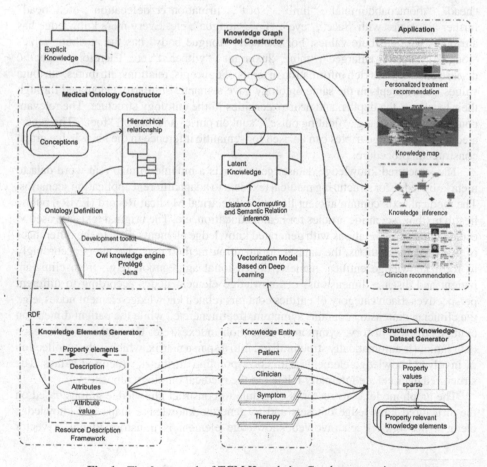

Fig. 1. The framework of TCM Knowledge Graph construction

ontology constructor, (2) a knowledge element generator, (3) a structured knowledge dataset generator, and (4) a graph model constructor.

The Medical ontology constructor is the module to construct medical domain ontology using explicit knowledge. Utilizing Natural Language Processing (NLP) technique, e.g., named entity recognition and text classification, we extract meta data from unstructured clinical texts. After that, The explicit knowledge including expert-defined traditional Chinese medicines, modern medical knowledge from clinical protocol guidelines and medical textbooks are acquired. According to the Chinese medicine terminology standards published by Chinese government, we generate a hierarchical structure as the base of the ontology by following the Resource Description Framework (RDF) and Ontology Web Language (OWL-Lite). The process is under the supervision of domain experts and assisted with an ontology edition tool Protégé[1].

The knowledge element generator is a module to generate knowledge triples containing meta knowledge attributes and relations. Here "meta knowledge" is an extensive notion including all concepts and their relations defined in RDF. For example, "inspection" associates with specific scope (related to human body parts) including "head", "thoracoabdominal", "limb", "sprit", "urination & defecation", etc. "head" further associates with "face", "eye", "lip", "tongue", etc. Every meta knowledge has attributes with attribute values. For example, "tongue body" has the attribute values "tough", "tender", "enlarged", "thin", "luxuriant", "withered", etc. Therefore, a specific disease ontology has rich information in terms of concepts, relations, attributes, attribute values. All concepts in the same ontology have semantic similarity calculated through their locations, the depths, and nearby densities in the ontology structure. The relevant concepts are closer, e.g., "floating pulse"-"sunken pulse" and "limb"-"foot". The generated meta knowledge triples can be used for semantic inference in the knowledge graph construction procedure.

The structured knowledge dataset generator is a module to map real word data to meta knowledge for structuring medical text data to adapt different application scenarios. The medical texts contain ancient literature, Electrical Medical Record (EMR), public health textbox, scientific articles for health education, etc. The original texts are used to establish mapping relations with generated knowledge elements. Due to the differences of practical applications, the dataset organization method may also alters accordingly to form knowledge entities, namely, dimensional aggregation (e.g., from clinician, patient and disease dimensions) of knowledge element nodes according to different perspectives. Each category of entities contains related knowledge element nodes, e.g., the clinician dimension contains symptom, treatment, etc., while the patient dimension contains disease history, symptoms, inspection indexes, etc. Using the module, each data sample is automatically structuralized into a sparse matrix, which is the +collection of involved knowledge elements with corresponding attributes structured values. The structured datasets are internally related to the medical ontology repository.

The graph model constructor is a module to construct knowledge graphs based on the structured knowledge datasets and to generate knowledge maps and knowledge element networks. Each involved knowledge element is transformed into a vector

---

[1] http://protege.stanford.edu/.

representation after the structured datasets goes through a vectorization model based on deep learning algorithms. To calculate the semantic distance and the inference of semantic relations, an unsupervised learning is applied to generate a knowledge map by calculating the distance among knowledge element vectors according to preset categories. The semantic inference refers to the prediction of correlations of knowledge elements based on the graph model, which returns the weighted directed complex network according to relation weights. The knowledge map reflects the latent correlation among knowledge elements, and the directed knowledge element complex network reflects the latent logical relation among knowledge elements, while the weight reflects the popularity degree of the logical rules. The entire construction process of the knowledge graph can be regarded as a process of discovering latent knowledge.

4   Experiments and Results

To evaluate the effectiveness of the framework in Traditional Chinese Medicine (TCM) knowledge graph construction, we use a publically available "Levis hypertension" Chinese clinical dataset [20], which contains 908 hypertension TCM cases. The dataset has rich case information and each case has 129 dimensions of diagnosis and symptoms including "inspection diagnosis" (望诊), "inquiry diagnosis" (问诊), "tongue diagnosis and palpation diagnosis" (舌脉) etc. After removing 22 cases because of diagnosis information missing, we obtain 886 cases eventually for the evaluation with ten-folder cross-validation. The summary of the dataset is shown in Table 1.

Table 1.   The summary of the hypertension TCM dataset.

Dataset	Feature dimensions	# of cases	Data type
Training set	129	797	*Boolean*
Testing set	129	89	*Boolean*
Total	129	886	*Boolean*

According to the standards of the syndrome of TCM (中医证候) [21], we manually extract major characteristics of TCM syndrome for each case and use them as gold reference labels, in which each case has 2 to 5 labels. The experiment on the dataset thus is converted to a multi-label classification problem. Part of the characteristics of TCM syndrome elements (证候要素) is listed in Table 2.

In order to optimize the iteration parameter β in the learning process, we use the ML-KNN algorithm [22] and RAKEL-SMO algorithm [23] on the training dataset. Using evaluation metrics including hamming loss, average precision, micro-averaged precision, micro-averaged F-measure, macro-averaged precision, macro-averaged F-measure, and micro-averaged AUC, the performances are presented in Fig. 2. The first of Fig. 2 shows that the ML-KNN algorithm ($k = 12$, $V = 0.1$) tends to be more stable when iteration β is greater than or equal to 75, while the second presents that the RAKEL-SMO algorithm ($S = 6$, $V = 0.1$) becomes stable when β is greater than or equal to 100. We therefore select the best iteration parameter β as 100.

Table 2. The summarized characteristics of the symptoms of Traditional Chinese Medicine

Categorized inquiry features	Clinical symptoms
Face	Facial flush, Red face, Dark pale complexion, Flushing, Pale white, A pale complexion, Pale complexion
Head	Empty pain of head, Dizziness, Head and eye distending pain, Headache, Fullness in head, Heavy sensation of head, Head with binding sensation, Vertigo
Eye	Red eye, Dry eye, Dizzy, Fullness in eye, Hypopsia, Blurred vision
Lip	Purple lips, Lip colorless, Dark lips
Ear	Eared, Deaf, Tinnitus
Thoracoabdominal & limb	Oppression in chest, Pectoralgia, Distention and fullness, Hypochondriac pain, Soreness of waist, Limb numbness, Leg soft, Ventosity, Soreness and weakness of knees

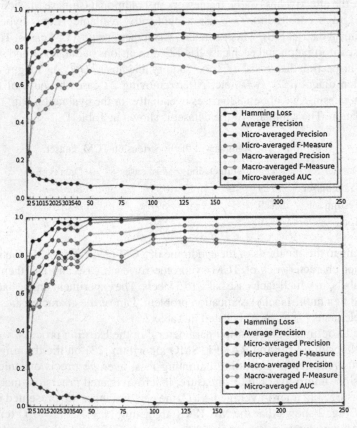

Fig. 2. The performance of ML-KNN and RAKEL-SMO algorithms with the increasing number of learning iterations

Due to difficulties to acquire entity relations corresponding to knowledge graph from unstructured texts directly, the annotation on texts to build a gold standard for the evaluation relation prediction by knowledge graph thus is infeasible. Therefore, we test the effectiveness of the constructed TCM knowledge graph by comparing the classification performance differences of machine learning algorithms with and without the knowledge graph. Using the exact same ML-KNN and RAKEL-SMO algorithms with the optimized iteration β, we take the converted vectors of meta knowledge from the TCM knowledge graph as features as "KG" regarding to "conventional" features using commonly used algorithms. In each experiment, ten-folder cross-validation evaluation was used on the testing dataset. The comparison result is reported in Table 3.

Table 3. The performance comparison with and without knowledge graph vectors as features.

Methods/Metrics	ML-KNN ($k = 12$, $V = 0.1$)			RAKEL-SMO ($S = 6$, $V = 0.1$)		
	Conventional	+KG	Change	Conventional	+KG	Change
Micro-averaged precision	0.717 ± 0.064	0.888 ± 0.022	23.8%	0.686 ± 0.057	0.945 ± 0.019	37.8%
Micro-averaged recall	0.489 ± 0.037	0.848 ± 0.019	73.4%	0.608 ± 0.051	0.988 ± 0.005	62.5%
Micro-averaged F-measure	0.581 ± 0.043	0.867 ± 0.017	49.2%	0.644 ± 0.051	0.966 ± 0.010	50.0%
Macro-averaged precision	0.376 ± 0.064	0.760 ± 0.032	102.1%	0.340 ± 0.050	0.861 ± 0.071	153.2%
Macro-averaged recall	0.289 ± 0.038	0.671 ± 0.041	132.2%	0.526 ± 0.054	0.881 ± 0.060	67.5%
Macro-averaged F-measure	0.303 ± 0.040	0.697 ± 0.034	130.0%	0.404 ± 0.052	0.868 ± 0.063	114.9%
Average precision	0.745 ± 0.048	0.946 ± 0.011	27.0%	0.755 ± 0.044	0.980 ± 0.007	29.8%
Mean average precision	0.385 ± 0.038	0.813 ± 0.047	111.2%	0.418 ± 0.045	0.908 ± 0.044	117.2%
Ranking loss	0.119 ± 0.021	0.022 ± 0.005	−81.5%	0.132 ± 0.026	0.006 ± 0.004	−95.5%
Logarithmic soss	4.626 ± 0.344	1.937 ± 0.227	−58.1%	14.06 ± 2.341	0.732 ± 0.275	−94.8%

From the results, the ML-KNN and RAkEL-SMO algorithms with conventional feature extraction strategy obtain an average precision of 0.745 ± 0.048 and 0.755 ± 0.044, respectively. By combining with the knowledge graph (+KG), the average precision is increased to 0.946 ± 0.011 and 0.980 ± 0.007 with an improvement of 27.0% and 29.8%, respectively. Similarly, the micro-averaged F-measure performance is increased from 0.581 ± 0.043 and 0.644 ± 0.051 to 0.867 ± 0.017 and 0.966 ± 0.010 with an improvement of 49.2% and 50.0%, while the macro-averaged F-Measure performance is increased from 0.303 ± 0.040 and 0.404 ± 0.052 to 0.697 ± 0.034 and 0.868 ± 0.063 with an improvement of 130.0% and 114.9%, respectively. The results on ranking loss and logarithmic metrics also show the usage of TCM knowledge graph significantly outperforming the conventional feature extraction, demonstrating that the constructed TCM knowledge graph can benefit the performance of machine learning algorithms on multi-label classification tasks.

5 Discussions

The constructed TCM knowledge graph can be visualized into dynamic map for clinicians to interactively observe the connections between concepts, for providing the references for the purpose of disease syndrome type summarization. On the other hand, the knowledge graph can generate complex network for reflecting the inferences between meta knowledge in the network. As shown in Fig. 3, the inferences are the edges representing the concept relations among concept nodes. All the edges have directions and weights, where the directions denote sequential relations, e.g., *X medicine treat Y disease*, *X disease has Y symptom*, etc. The weight values of the edges denotes the strengthness and weakness of the relations. The weights can be learned and adjusted for helping clinicians in observing and filtering the relations to obtain relation patterns.

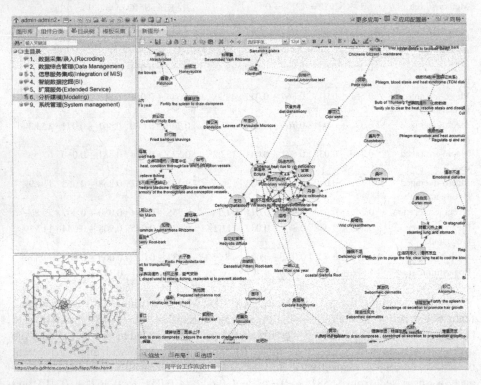

Fig. 3. The visualization of the TCM knowledge graph for clinicians to operate interactively

The constructed TCM knowledge graph can also be potentially utilized for decision making assistant. We develop a system named as "Intelligent profile analysis and recommendation based on TCM knowledge graph", as shown in Fig. 4. The decision making assistant in the system mainly has the following steps: (1) retrieve and filter the meta knowledge in the knowledge graph according to the symptoms, observational data, lab test, etc.; (2) observe the distributions of the attributes of diagnosis, medicine, prognosis in the knowledge graph and import the meta nodes into the vectorization model as described in the framework for structuring the data; (3) generate a knowledge map network according to the vector representations; (4) observe the results of network clustering and analyze the references for initial patient diagnosis and treatment strategies; (5) obtain assisted decision making references of patient treatment strategies according to the semantic inference among the meta knowledge such as the symptoms and lab test values of the patients.

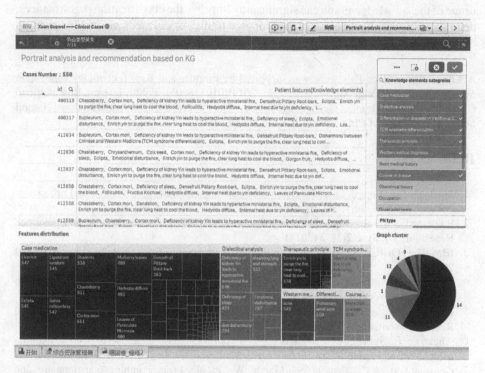

Fig. 4. The user interface of a developed system named as "Intelligent profile analysis and recommendation based on TCM knowledge graph" for decision making assistant

Until now, the system based on the TCM knowledge graph has been applied to the analysis of more than 1000 ancient Chinese medicine books, and the information extraction from the medical records for more than ten TCM departments in provincial hospitals. Particularly, the system has been used to serve for 5 national/provincial level famous TCM experts in the summarization of their clinical cases. In short, the system not only implements the TCM knowledge retrieval and network analysis but also provides the summarization and visualization of famous TCM experts through the knowledge discovery from their related EMR text data. We believe the system could further benefit the interactions among TCM clinicians and even the knowledge accumulation for public health knowledge spread.

6 Conclusions

Targeting at medical knowledge graph construction, this paper proposes a framework for automated Traditional Chinese Medicine knowledge graph construction from existing clinical texts. The framework consists of four major modules. Based on a standard dataset containing 886 patient cases, the evaluation results present that the usage of the knowledge graph can significantly improve the classification performances, demonstrating the effectiveness of the proposed framework in medical knowledge graph construction.

Acknowledgements. This work was supported by Frontier and Key Technology Innovation Special Grant of Guangdong Province (No. 2014B010118005), Public Interest Research and Capability Building Grant of Guangdong Province (No. 2014A020221039), and National Natural Science Foundation of China (No. 61772146 & 61403088).

References

1. Jameson, J.L., Longo, D.L.: Precision medicine-personalized, problematic, and promising. Obstetr. Gynecol. Surv. **70**(10), 612–614 (2015)
2. Raghupathi, W., Raghupathi, V.: Big data analytics in healthcare: promise and potential. Health Inf. Sci. Syst. **2**(1), 3 (2014)
3. IBM-The FOUR V's of Big Data. http://www-01.ibm.com/software/data/bigdata/. Accessed 2017
4. Sagiroglu, S., Sinanc, D.: Big data: a review. In: Proceedings of International Conference on Collaboration Technologies and Systems, pp. 42–47 (2013)
5. Belle, A., Thiagarajan, R., Soroushmehr, S., et al.: Big Data Analytics in Healthcare. BioMed Research International (2015)
6. Alickovic, E., Subasi, A.: Medical decision support system for diagnosis of heart arrhythmia using DWT and random forests classifier. J. Med. Syst. **40**(4), 1–12 (2016)
7. Constantinou, A.C., Fenton, N., Marsh, W., et al.: From complex questionnaire and interviewing data to intelligent Bayesian network models for medical decision support. Artif. Intell. Med. **67**, 75–93 (2016)
8. Woosley, R., Whyte, J., Mohamadi, A., et al.: Medical decision support systems and therapeutics: the role of autopilots. Clin. Pharmacol. Ther. **99**(2), 161–164 (2016)
9. Cambria, E., Olsher, D., Rajagopal, D.: SenticNet 3: a common and common-sense knowledge base for cognition-driven sentiment analysis. In: Proceedings of Twenty-Eighth AAAI Conference on Artificial Intelligence (2014)
10. Mirzaa, G.M., Millen, K.J., Barkovich, A.J., et al.: The developmental brain disorders database (DBDB): a curated neurogenetics knowledge base with clinical and research applications. Am. J. Med. Genet. Part A **164**(6), 1503–1511 (2014)
11. Taglang, G.D., Jackson, B.: Use of "big data" in drug discovery and clinical trials. Gynecol. Oncol. **141**(1), 17–23 (2016)
12. Vicini, P., Fields, O., Lai, E., et al.: Precision medicine in the age of big data: the present and future role of large-scale unbiased sequencing in drug discovery and development. Clin. Pharmacol. Ther. **99**(2), 198–207 (2016)
13. Holzinger, A.: Trends in interactive knowledge discovery for personalized medicine: cognitive science meets machine learning. IEEE Intell. Inform. Bull. **15**(1), 6–14 (2014)

14. Kim, D., Joung, J.G., Sohn, K.A., et al.: Knowledge boosting: a graph-based integration approach with multi-omics data and genomic knowledge for cancer clinical outcome prediction. J. Am. Med. Inform. Assoc. **22**(1), 109–120 (2015)
15. Kamsu-Foguem, B., Tchuenté-Foguem, G., Foguem, C.: Using conceptual graphs for clinical guidelines representation and knowledge visualization. Inf. Syst. Front. **16**(4), 571–589 (2014)
16. Zhang, D., Xie, Y., Li, M., et al.: Construction of knowledge graph of traditional Chinese medicine based on the ontology. Technol. Intell. Eng. **3**(1), 8 (2017)
17. Yu, T., Li, J., Yu, Q., et al.: Knowledge graph for TCM health preservation: design, construction, and applications. Artif. Intell. Med. **77**, 48–52 (2017)
18. Shi, L., Li, S., Yang, X., et al.: Semantic Health Knowledge Graph: Semantic Integration of Heterogeneous Medical Knowledge and Services. BioMed Research International (2017)
19. Mikolov, T., Kombrink, S., Deoras, A., et al.: RNNLM-recurrent neural network language modeling toolkit. In: Proceedings of the 2011 ASRU Workshop, pp. 196–201 (2011)
20. Ou, A., Lin, X., Li, G., et al.: LEVIS: a hypertension dataset in traditional Chinese medicine. In: Proceedings of Bioinformatics and Biomedicine (BIBM), pp. 192–197 (2013)
21. State Administration of Traditional Chinese Medicine of People's Republic of China: Clinic terminology of traditional Chinese medical diagnosis and treatment–Syndromes. Standards Press of China, Beijing, GB/T 16751.2–1997 (1997)
22. Zhang, M.L., Zhou, Z.H.: ML-KNN: a lazy learning approach to multi-label learning. Pattern Recogn. **40**(7), 2038–2048 (2007)
23. Sorower, M.S.: A Literature Survey on Algorithms for Multi-label Learning. Oregon State University, Corvallis (2010)

Author Index

Printed in the United States
By Bookmasters